# Other titles in this series

# COLORADO

## YOUR CAR-CAMPING GUIDE TO SCENIC BEAUTY, THE SOUNDS OF NATURE, AND AN ESCAPE FROM CIVILIZATION

### Fifth Edition

## KIM LIPKER and JOHNNY MOLLOY

**MENASHA RIDGE PRESS**

BIRMINGHAM, ALABAMA

*For John Bland, who got it all started.* —JM

## Best Tent Camping: Colorado

Copyright © 2012 by Johnny Molloy and Kim Lipker
All rights reserved
Printed in the United States of America
Published by Menasha Ridge Press
Distributed by the Publishers Group West
Fifth edition, first printing

ISBN: 978-0-89732-990-3
eISBN: 978-0-89732-991-0

CATALOGING-IN-PUBLICATION DATA IS AVAILABLE FROM THE LIBRARY OF CONGRESS

Cover design by Scott McGrew
Cover photo by J. C. Leacock/Alamy
Text design by Ian Szymkowiak/Palace Press International, Inc.
Cartography by Steve Jones, Kim Lipker, and Johnny Molloy
Indexing by Rich Carlson

Menasha Ridge Press
P.O. Box 43673
Birmingham, Alabama 35243
**www.menasharidge.com**

# TABLE OF CONTENTS

# COLORADO CAMPGROUND AWARDS

## BEST FOR PRIVACY

## BEST FOR SPACIOUSNESS

## BEST FOR QUIET

## BEST FOR SECURITY

## BEST FOR CLEANLINESS

## BEST FOR WHEELCHAIRS

# ACKNOWLEDGMENTS

**I** WOULD LIKE TO THANK JOHNNY MOLLOY; the folks at Menasha Ridge Press; my friends and my family; and the helpful folks at the National Park Service, the USDA Forest Service, and the Colorado State Parks.

—*Kim Lipker*

**T** HANKS TO THE FOLLOWING FOR THEIR help with the original editions of the guide: Joe Mayer, Sam Berry, Becky Anderson, Kate Brannan, Paul Welschinger, Susan Webster, Margaret Albrecht, Bryan Delay, James Herbaugh, Pat Molloy, Bill Armstrong, Keith Stinnett, Bryan Hatfield, Michael and Nan Wolfenbarger, Nelle Molloy, Larry of Castle Rock; Beverly, Wilbert, and Craig Spieker of Castle Rock, who made me feel at home; Regi Roberts, John Cox, and David Zaczyk, master of the semicolon.

—*Johnny Molloy*

# PREFACE

**OH, WHAT A JOY IT WAS** to research this book! In the beginning, the task of finding the 50 best campgrounds in Colorado seemed daunting, for there are hundreds of campgrounds located among the millions of acres of national- and state-forest land, national parks and monuments, and other public lands. But the months of exploring Colorado's varied landscape turned into a journey through a scenic wonderland. The Rockies come to mind first, where craggy, snow-covered mountains tower over verdant meadows, cool alpine lakes reflect deep forests and cobalt skies, and snow-fed mountain streams crash down narrow valleys. But there are other sides of Colorado: the amazing cliff dwellings of Mesa Verde, the chasm of the Black Canyon of the Gunnison, the alluring reservoirs of the plains, the immense Great Sand Dunes backed against the Sangre de Cristo Range, the white water of the Arkansas River, the red-rock country of the Uncompahgre Plateau, and more.

After seeing this tremendous variation, I wanted the reader to enjoy these sights while having a great camping experience. I toured the state's natural and historic features by day, then typed up on-site reports from the nearby camps where I stayed.

Each day's experience left me looking forward to the next day, to see if I could find campgrounds to match the beauty of the landscape. Spells of cold and rain and wrong turns and long drives to campgrounds that failed to make the book could not overwhelm the sense of awe I felt while surveying the real Colorado. The subject material overwhelmed the actual physical process of finding the best campgrounds. In other words, researching Colorado was a blast!

And it can be for you, too, pitching your tent at 3,500 feet in the plains or 12,000 feet in the mountains, and just about every elevation and situation in between. Here, you can relax in attractive settings. Beyond the campgrounds you can hike canyons, climb "fourteeners," raft wild rivers, fish remote trout streams, mountain bike tabletop mesas, boat reservoirs, go caving, and recall Colorado's history. Combine this book and a slice of your precious time, then do a little exploring of your own.

*—Johnny Molloy*

## A Note about the Fifth Edition

Revising something that is otherwise perfect is, again, both an honor and a daunting task. I was approached as a Rocky Mountain expert to update existing profiles, delete old campgrounds, and add new ones. We also reorganized the book according to more commonly known regions (around these parts, at least), refined the maps, and wrote a more thorough introduction to tent camping—all while keeping the same friendly tone and accuracy for which Johnny Molloy is known. We hope you'll like the changes, and we encourage you to get out and find your favorite "room with a view" in Colorado.

*—Kim Lipker*

# ABOUT THE AUTHORS

**J**OHNNY MOLLOY IS AN OUTDOOR WRITER based in Johnson City, Tennessee. Born in Memphis, he moved to Knoxville in 1980 to attend the University of Tennessee.

During his college years, he developed a love of the natural world that has since become the primary focus of his life.

It all started on a backpacking foray into the Great Smoky Mountains National Park. That first trip was a disaster; nevertheless, Johnny discovered an affinity for the outdoors that would lead him to backpack and canoe-camp throughout the United States over the next 25 years. Today, he averages 150 nights out per year.

After graduating from UT with a degree in Economics, Johnny spent an ever-increasing amount of time in the wild, becoming more skilled in a variety of environments. Friends enjoyed his adventure stories; one even suggested that he write a book. He pursued that idea and soon parlayed his love of the outdoors into an occupation.

The results of his efforts are more than 40 books. These include hiking, camping, paddling, and other comprehensive guidebooks, as well as books on true outdoor adventures. Johnny has also written for numerous publications and websites. He continues to write and travel extensively to all four corners of the United States, exploring a variety of outdoor activities. For the latest on Johnny, please visit **johnnymolloy.com.**

**K**IM LIPKER GREW UP IN COLORADO loving the outdoors from an early age. She is the author of three other guidebooks for Menasha Ridge Press, *60 Hikes within 60 Miles: Denver and Boulder, Day & Overnight Hikes in Rocky Mountain National Park,* and *Smart and Savvy Hiking for Women.* She also wrote *The Unofficial Guide to Bed & Breakfasts and Country Inns in the Rockies* (Hungry Minds). In addition to writing books, Kim works for two local nonprofits. She was an expert contributor for Away.com, a division of Orbitz. She contributes features, ratings, and reviews for Away.com, covering parks, active sports, and outdoor adventures in the Rocky Mountains and Hawaii.

Considered an expert on the Rocky Mountains by her guidebook peers, Kim has been at the writing thing for a while, having had her first news article published at age 12 and later earning a journalism degree from the University of Missouri–Columbia. Kim lives in Fort Collins, Colorado, with her three children.

# INTRODUCTION

**W**ELCOME TO THE FIFTH EDITION OF *Best Tent Camping: Colorado*. If you're new to tent camping or even if you're a seasoned camper, take a few minutes to read the following introduction. We explain how this book is organized and how to use it.

## THE OVERVIEW MAP AND OVERVIEW-MAP KEY

Use the overview map on the inside front cover to assess the exact location of each campground. The campground's number appears not only on the overview map but also on the map key facing the overview map, in the table of contents, and on the profile's first page.

The book is organized by region as indicated in the table of contents. A map legend that details the symbols found on the campground layout maps appears on the inside back cover.

## CAMPGROUND-LAYOUT MAPS

Each profile contains a detailed campground layout map that provides an overhead look at campground sites, internal roads, facilities, and other key items. Each campground entrance's GPS coordinates are included with each profile.

## GPS CAMPGROUND-ENTRANCE COORDINATES

This book includes the GPS coordinates for each campground entrance. Topographic maps show latitude–longitude as well as UTM grid lines. The survey datum used to arrive at the coordinates in this book is WGS84 (versus NAD27 or WGS83). For readers who own a GPS unit, whether handheld or onboard a vehicle, the latitude–longitude may be entered into the GPS unit. Just make sure your GPS unit is set to navigate using WGS84 datum. Now you can navigate directly to the campground.

However, readers can easily find all campgrounds in this book by using the directions given and the campground layout map, which shows at least one major road leading into the area. But for those who enjoy using the latest GPS technology to navigate, the necessary data has been provided.

## THE CAMPGROUND PROFILE

In addition to maps each profile contains a concise but informative narrative of the campground, as well as individual sites. This descriptive text is enhanced with at-a-glance ratings and information, GPS-based trailhead coordinates, and accurate driving directions that lead you from a major road to the parking area most convenient to the trailhead. On the first page of each profile is a ratings box.

# THE RATING SYSTEM

This book includes a rating system for Colorado's 50 best tent campgrounds. Six campground attributes—beauty, privacy, spaciousness, quiet, security, and cleanliness—are ranked using a five-star system. A low rating in one or two areas, especially privacy and spaciousness, was not necessarily grounds for exclusion from this book. In some cases, the nature of the terrain just doesn't allow for big, private sites, yet the campground still may be well worth a visit. This system should help you find what you are looking for.

## Beauty

In judging beauty, we took into account both what the general area has to offer as well as the campground. The most beautiful campgrounds have sites that you just don't want to leave and locations with easy access to breathtaking scenery.

## Privacy

Privacy is determined by how much your neighbors can pay attention to what you are doing and you to what they are doing. The best campgrounds have plenty of green space (shrubs and trees) between adjoining sites, as well as staggered sites (that is, the entrance to the site across the road is not directly opposite yours).

## Spaciousness

While this category contributes to the amount of privacy you have, it refers mostly to how much space you have to move around in. The sites at some campgrounds are surprisingly large—to the point of overkill; others are incredibly small.

## Quiet

Our evaluations were influenced to a great extent by the presence of RVs and the kinds of visitors a park tends to get (campgrounds near urban areas, for example, usually are a bit noisy, as are those that cater to families with children). We also considered the extent to which you could get away from the fray at a particular campground. You can expect some variation within our ratings based on whether you visit a campground during the week or on a weekend; on holiday weekends, all bets are off.

## Security

With few exceptions, we've found Colorado campgrounds to be very safe and secure, due largely to the presence of campground hosts and park rangers making the rounds. The only places at which we felt security might be compromised were those remote campgrounds that saw few visitors and had no host or ranger on duty.

## Cleanliness

Our judgments were based on the presence and remnants of past campers around the campsite (trash, tent stakes, burned logs, etc.) and on the restroom facilities. We did take into account that primitive toilets tend to be a little less tidy than modern facilities, although there seemed to us to be little reason for either to be a mess.

# WEATHER

We must stress that the weather in Colorado can change every ten minutes. Be prepared for anything: sun, snow, flash flood, lightning, and hail. Start by knowing the weather forecast and the road conditions; then pack smart. It can be a lovely day in Denver, but a campground may be inaccessible due to blizzard conditions. You must be prepared, and you should consider carrying a hiking card (CORSAR, discussed on the next page). If you need to be rescued, these cards can save your life and your pocketbook.

## Climate Overview

Semiarid            Short springs
Dry summers        Mild winters except in the mountains

| MEAN TEMPERATURE BY MONTH: DENVER AREA | | | | | |
|---|---|---|---|---|---|
| | JAN | FEB | MAR | APR | MAY | JUN |
| HIGH | 43 | 47 | 52 | 62 | 71 | 81 |
| LOW | 16 | 20 | 26 | 35 | 44 | 52 |
| | JUL | AUG | SEP | OCT | NOV | DEC |
| HIGH | 88 | 86 | 77 | 66 | 53 | 45 |
| LOW | 59 | 57 | 48 | 36 | 25 | 17 |

It is hard to generalize the climate and the altitude throughout Colorado, but we can tell you that what you pack and how you deal with the altitude can make or break a camping trip.

The Rockies' rugged and varied geography creates a number of weather zones. Whatever the region, whatever the season, be sure to dress in layers. In the summer, expect warm days and cool evenings. Bring shorts, hiking boots, a sweater, and a weatherproof jacket. In the winter, bring snow gear for the mountains and warm outerwear for elsewhere.

## Altitude Sickness

Nothing ruins an outing more often than the body's resistance to altitude adjustment. The illness is usually characterized by vomiting, loss of breath, extreme headache, lightheadedness, sleeplessness, and an overall sick feeling. Our advice: take it easy. When traveling to a higher altitude, give your body a day or two to adjust to where there is less oxygen, hotter sun, and less air pressure. Drink plenty of water and lay off the alcohol and cigarettes. Wear sunglasses and sunscreen. It's that easy. (As always, if serious symptoms persist, locate the nearest emergency room or call 911.)

## Lightning and Tornadoes

Violent storms are common in June, July, and August. If you are caught in a lightning storm above treeline, stay off ridgetops, spread out if you are in a group and squat or sit on a foam pad with your feet together. Keep away from rock outcroppings and isolated trees. If someone has been struck, be prepared to use CPR to help restore breathing and heartbeat.

In the event of a tornado (they are extremely common in the eastern portion of Colorado), immediately seek shelter. If you are in an open field, lie down in the nearest ditch.

# CORSAR

The Colorado Outdoor Recreation Search and Rescue Card (CORSAR) may be purchased at most outdoor shops, such as REI. You can buy a one-year card for $3 or spend $12 and buy a five-year card. CORSAR is not insurance—it does not pay for medical transportation, which may include helicopter flights or ground ambulance. The card does allow reimbursement to county sheriffs for costs included on a mission. These expenses can include mileage, meals, equipment, gasoline, and rental fees (horses, ATVs, aircraft) for vehicles used in the search. It says right on the CORSAR information that "you have helped ensure that trained and well-equipped search and rescue teams will respond should you become lost or in need of rescue and they will not have to incur undue expense due to your emergency."

# FIRST-AID KIT

A typical first-aid kit may contain more items than you might think necessary. These are just the basics. Prepackaged kits in waterproof bags are available (Atwater Carey and Adventure Medical make a variety of such kits). As a preventive measure, take along sunscreen and insect repellent. Even though there are quite a few items in the following list, they do pack down into a small space:

Ace bandages or Spenco joint wraps

Adhesive bandages

Antibiotic ointment (Neosporin or the generic equivalent)

Antiseptic or disinfectant, such as Betadine or hydrogen peroxide

Aspirin or acetaminophen

Benadryl or the generic equivalent, diphenhydramine (in case of allergic reactions)

Butterfly-closure bandages

Epinephrine in a prefilled syringe (for people known to have severe allergic reactions to such things as bee stings)

Gauze (one roll)

Gauze compresses (six 4 x 4–inch pads)

Matches or pocket lighter

Moleskin or Spenco 2nd Skin

Waterproof first-aid tape

Whistle (it's more effective in signaling rescuers than your voice is)

# ANIMAL AND PLANT HAZARDS

## Black Bears

There are no definite rules about what to do if you meet a bear. In most cases the bear will detect you first and leave. If you do encounter a bear, here are some suggestions from the National Park Service:

• Stay calm.

• Move away, talking loudly to let the bear discover your presence.

• Back away while facing the bear.

• Avoid eye contact.

• Give the bear plenty of room to escape; bears will rarely attack unless they are threatened or provoked.

• Don't run or make sudden movements; running will provoke the bear and you can not outrun a bear.

- Do not attempt to climb trees to escape bears, especially a black bear. The bear will pull you down by the foot.
- Fight back if you are attacked. Black bears have been driven away when people have fought back with rocks, sticks, binoculars, and even their bare hands.
- Be grateful that it's not a grizzly bear.

## Mountain Lions

Lion attacks on people are rare, with fewer than 12 fatalities in 100 years. Based on observations by people who have come in contact with mountain lions, some patterns are beginning to emerge. Here are more suggestions from the National Park Service:

- Stay calm.
- Talk firmly to the lion.
- Move slowly.
- Back up or stop; never run because lions will chase and attack.
- Raise your arms. If you are wearing a sweater or coat; open it and hold it wide.
- Pick up children and make them appear larger.
- If the lion becomes aggressive, throw rocks and large objects at it. This is the time to convince the lion that you are not prey and that you are a danger to them.
- Never crouch down, or turn your back to retrieve said items.
- Fight back and try to remain standing if you are attacked.

## Ticks

Ticks like to hang out in the brush that grows around campsites and along trails. Their numbers seem to explode in the hot summer months, but you should be tick-aware during all months of the year. Ticks, which are arthropods and not insects, need a host to feast on in order to reproduce. The ticks that light onto you will be very small, sometimes so tiny that you won't be able to spot them. Primarily of two varieties, deer ticks and dog ticks, both need a few hours of actual attachment before they can transmit any disease they may harbor. Ticks may settle in shoes, socks, hats, and may take several hours to actually latch on. The best strategy is to visually check yourself a couple of times a day, especially if you've gone out for a walk in the woods. Ticks that haven't attached are easily removed, but not easily killed. If you pick off a tick in the woods, just toss it aside. If you find one on your body at camp, you may want to dispatch it (otherwise, it may find you again). For ticks that are embedded, removal with tweezers is best.

**RATTLESNAKE**

## Snakes

Spend some time in Colorado and you may be surprised by the variety of snakes in the area. Most snake encounters will be with garter snakes, water snakes, and bull snakes

(while not venomous, they are rather large and scary looking). The only venomous snake in the region is the rattlesnake. Rattler sightings are very common. A good rule of thumb is to give rattlers a wide berth and leave them alone. In the chance that you are bitten by a rattlesnake stay calm and get help immediately.

### Poison Ivy

Recognizing poison ivy and avoiding contact with it is the most effective way to prevent the painful, itchy rashes associated with these plants. In the West, poison ivy is found as a small plant with three leaflets to a leaf. Remember "leaves of three, let them be." Urushiol,

**POISON IVY**

the oil in the sap of these plants, is responsible for the rash. Usually within 12 to 14 hours of exposure (but sometimes much later), raised lines and/or blisters will appear, accompanied by a terrible itch. Refrain from scratching because bacteria under fingernails can cause infection and you will spread the rash to other parts of your body. Wash and dry the rash thoroughly, applying calamine lotion or another product to help dry the rash. If itching or blistering is severe, seek medical attention. Remember that oil-contaminated clothes, pets, or hiking gear can easily cause an irritating rash on you or someone else, so wash not only any exposed parts of your body but also clothes, gear, and pets.

### Mosquitoes

Although it's not a common occurrence, individuals can become infected with the West Nile virus by being bitten by an infected mosquito. Culex mosquitoes, the primary variety that can transmit West Nile virus to humans, thrive in urban rather than natural areas. They lay their eggs in stagnant water and can breed in any standing water that remains for more than five days.

Most people infected with West Nile virus have no symptoms of illness, but some may become ill, usually 3 to 15 days after being bitten. In Colorado, August and September are the high-risk periods for West Nile virus. At this time of year—and anytime you expect mosquitoes to be buzzing around—you may want to wear protective clothing such as long sleeves, long pants, and socks. Loose-fitting, light-colored clothing is best. Spray clothing with insect repellent. Remember to follow the instructions on the repellent carefully, and take extra care with children.

## TIPS FOR A HAPPY CAMPING TRIP

There is nothing worse than a bad camping trip, especially since it is so easy to have a great time. To assist with making your outing a happy one, here are some pointers:

- **RESERVE YOUR SITE AHEAD OF TIME,** especially if it's a weekend, a holiday, or if the campground is wildly popular. Many prime campgrounds require at least a six-month lead time on reservations. Check before you go.

- **PICK YOUR CAMPING BUDDIES WISELY.** A family trip is pretty straightforward, but you may want to consider including grumpy Uncle Fred who does not like bugs, sunshine, or

marshmallows. After you know who is going, make sure that everyone is on the same page regarding expectations of difficulty, sleeping arrangements, and food requirements.

- **DON'T DUPLICATE EQUIPMENT** such as cooking pots and lanterns among campers in your party. Carry what you need to have a good time, but don't turn the trip into a major moving experience.

- **DRESS APPROPRIATELY FOR THE SEASON.** Educate yourself on the highs and lows of the specific area you plan to visit. It may be warm at night in the summer in your backyard, but up in the mountains it will be quite chilly.

- **PITCH YOUR TENT ON A LEVEL SURFACE,** preferably one that is covered with leaves, pine straw, or grass. Pitch your tent on a tarp or specially designed footprint to thwart ground moisture and to protect the tent floor. Do a little site maintenance such as picking up small rocks and sticks that can damage your tent floor and make sleep uncomfortable. If you have a separate tent rain fly but don't need it, keep it rolled up at the base of the tent in case it starts raining at midnight.

- **IF YOU ARE NOT USED TO SLEEPING ON THE GROUND,** take a sleeping pad with you. Take one that is full-length and thicker than you think you might need. This will not only keep your hips from aching on hard ground, but will also help keep you warm.

- **IF YOU ARE NOT HIKING INTO A PRIMITIVE CAMPSITE**, there is no real need to skimp on food due to weight. Plan tasty meals and bring everything you will need to prepare, cook, eat, and clean up the mess.

- **IF YOU'RE PRONE TO USING THE BATHROOM MULTIPLE TIMES AT NIGHT,** you should plan ahead. Leaving a warm sleeping bag and stumbling around in the dark to find the restroom, whether it be an outhouse, a fully plumbed facility, or just the woods, is second best. Keep a flashlight and any other accoutrements you may need by the tent door and know exactly where to head in the dark.

- **STANDING DEAD TREES AND STORM-DAMAGED LIVING TREES** can pose a real hazard to tent campers. These trees may have loose or broken limbs that could fall at any time. When choosing a spot to rest or a backcountry campsite, look up.

## CAMPING ETIQUETTE

Camping experiences can vary wildly depending on a variety of factors such as weather, preparedness, fellow campers, and time of year. Here are a few tips on how to create good vibes with fellow campers and wildlife you encounter.

- **OBTAIN ALL PERMITS AND AUTHORIZATION AS REQUIRED.** Make sure you check in, pay your fee, and mark your site as directed. Don't make the mistake of grabbing a seemingly empty site that looks more appealing than your site. It could be reserved. If you are unhappy with the site you've selected, check with the campground host for other options.

- **LEAVE ONLY FOOTPRINTS.** Be sensitive to the ground beneath you. Be sure to place all garbage in designated receptacles or pack it out if none is available. No one likes to see the trash someone else has left behind.

- **NEVER SPOOK ANIMALS.** It's common for animals to wander through campsites, where they may be accustomed to the presence of humans (and our food). An unannounced approach, a sudden movement, or a loud noise startles most animals. A surprised animal can be dangerous to you, to others, and to themselves. Give them plenty of space.

- **PLAN AHEAD.** Know your equipment, your ability, and the area in which you are camping—and prepare accordingly. Be self-sufficient at all times; carry necessary supplies for changes in weather or other conditions. A well-executed trip is a satisfaction to you and to others.

- **BE COURTEOUS** to other campers, hikers, bikers, and others you encounter. If you run into the owner of a large RV, don't panic. Just wave, feign eye contact, and then walk away slowly.

- **STRICTLY FOLLOW THE CAMPGROUND'S RULES** regarding the building of fires. Never burn trash. Trash smoke smells horrible and trash debris in a fire pit or grill is unsightly.

## BACKCOUNTRY-CAMPING ADVICE

Be sure to check if a permit is required before entering the backcountry to camp and always strive to practice low-impact camping. Adhere to the adages "Pack it in, pack it out" and "Take only pictures, leave only footprints." Practice "leave no trace" camping ethics while in the backcountry.

Open fires are permitted except during dry times when the Forest Service may issue a fire ban. Backpacking stoves are strongly encouraged. You are required to hang your food from bears and other animals in order to minimize human impact on wildlife—avoid their introduction to and dependence on human food. Wildlife learns to associate backpacks and backpackers with easy food sources, thereby influencing its behavior. Make sure you have about 40 feet of thin but sturdy rope to properly secure your food. Ideally, you should throw your rope over a stout limb that extends ten or more feet above ground. Make sure the rope hangs at least five feet away from the tree trunk.

Solid human waste must be buried in a hole at least three inches deep and at least 200 feet away from trails and water sources; a trowel is basic backpacking equipment.

Following the above guidelines will increase your chances for a pleasant, safe, and low-impact interaction with nature.

## VENTURING AWAY FROM THE CAMPGROUND

If you go for a hike, bike, or other excursion into the boondocks, here are some tips:

- **ALWAYS CARRY FOOD AND WATER,** whether you are planning to go overnight or not. Food will give you energy, help keep you warm, and sustain you in an emergency situation until help arrives. You never know if you will have a stream nearby when you become thirsty. Bring potable water or treat water before drinking it from a stream. Boil or filter all found water before drinking it.

- **STAY ON DESIGNATED TRAILS.** Most hikers get lost when they leave the path. Even on the most clearly marked trails, there is usually a point where you have to stop and consider which direction to head. If you become disoriented, don't panic. As soon as you think you may be off-track, stop, assess your current direction, and then retrace your steps back to the point where you went awry. If you become absolutely unsure of how to continue, return to your vehicle the way you came in. Should you become completely lost and have no idea of how to return to the trailhead, remaining in place along the trail and waiting for help is most often the best option for adults and always the best option for children.

- **BE ESPECIALLY CAREFUL WHEN CROSSING STREAMS.** Whether you are fording the stream or crossing on a log, make every step count. If you have any doubt about maintaining your

balance on a foot log, go ahead and ford the stream instead. When fording a stream, use a trekking pole or stout stick for balance and face upstream as you cross. If a stream seems too deep to ford, turn back. Whatever is on the other side is not worth risking your life.

- **BE CAREFUL AT OVERLOOKS.** While these areas may provide spectacular views, they are potentially hazardous. Stay back from the edge of outcrops and be absolutely sure of your footing; a misstep can mean a nasty and possibly fatal fall.

- **KNOW THE SYMPTOMS OF HYPOTHERMIA.** Shivering and forgetfulness are the two most common indicators of this insidious killer. Hypothermia can occur at any elevation, even in the summer, especially when the hiker is wearing lightweight cotton clothing. If symptoms arise, get the victim shelter, hot liquids, and dry clothes or a dry sleeping bag.

- **TAKE ALONG YOUR BRAIN.** A cool, calculating mind is the single most important piece of equipment you'll ever need on the trail. Think before you act. Watch your step. Plan ahead. Avoiding accidents before they happen is the best recipe for a rewarding and relaxing hike.

# KIM'S TIPS FOR CAMPING WITH KIDS . . .

Camping with children can be a great way to introduce the young to the outdoors. It's also wonderful exercise and an even better family-bonding experience. It's time away from laundry, cell phones, and school—just you and the kids and nature.

## What to Bring

Packing for the kids is much like packing for the parents. Be sure each camper has the USDA Forest Service's "ten essentials": map, compass, water, knife, waterproof matches, high-energy food, suitable extra clothing (such as rain gear), mirror, first-aid kit, and whistle.

Consider packing my list of additional "ten kid essentials" for the tent: your child's favorite wholesome snack, juice, sunglasses, sunscreen, baby wipes, kid's trail map, kid's magnifying glass, scavenger-hunt cards, cuddle buddy, and permanent markers.

Be sure everyone is dressed for the weather. For hot or cold days, the rule is to dress in layers. All children need to have one proper pair of socks and one proper pair of shoes. Be sure there is no cotton in the socks, since cotton retains moisture and helps create blisters. Instead, buy child-sized wool socks and nylon liners—there are many different weights and variations for any condition.

Each child needs a sleeping bag that will fit his or her body type and provide warmth at night. Do your research on sizes and temperature ratings. (Don't cave in and get the Barbie sleeping bag little Susie really wants. Save that for slumber parties indoors.)

## Safety Considerations

Children should be taught from the get-go that they must stay within eyesight of an adult. They are to never run off. Not only can they get lost or injured, they can cause damage to the ecosystem. Teach your kids to treat the outdoors kindly, and the outdoors will repay the favor. Also teach children to stay where they are if they get lost. Many children relate to hugging a tree when lost—instruct them to find one, hold on, and blow their whistle. Three whistle blows is the standard distress signal, which indicates, "I am lost" or "I need

help." Never let kids go near steep cliffs and other drop-off areas. Rules about rivers and other water sources and climbing on accessible rocks must be addressed as well. (My rule is "No!")

Always teach outdoor etiquette: Leave no trace, pick up after others who do not, and don't pick or pull anything. And of course, leaves of three, let them be.

## Keep It Fun

Before you leave home, have the kids help make a special kid-friendly map of the campground area that they can keep in their bag. Making maps helps teach direction and creativity. Create a kid-friendly legend that has items like waterfalls, trails, trees, or tents. Have the child mark interesting points of interest while they are camping.

Toy stores are home to many camping or backyard camping things such as kids' magnifying glasses. A magnifying glass can be used to identify plants, insects, minerals in rocks, and flowers.

Make scavenger-hunt cards to use on any hike away from the campground (or in the area around the campground). A stack of index cards works fine. Have your child cut camping-related items from used magazines and paste them on each card. If your child can draw, this works as well. Write the name under the item and bring as many as you want. You can prolong your scavenger hunt cards throughout the summer by simply marking each item that you see on the back. It's fun to have a trump card that could be tucked away for special sightings: bull snake, lost watch, or an abandoned sock. Bring a permanent marker to take notes on your cards—some may even want to laminate their cards.

Play games like "I Spy," try bird-watching, look for animal tracks, or simply count rocks in the campground. The key is to play games that encourage children to observe their surroundings.

Assign a camping leader (or mountain leader as we call it) and have that child guide the camping trip. Have them plan the menu, decide when meals will be served, and even let them pick bedtime (don't worry; most campers go to bed when the sun goes down). Have your child invite a friend, which helps your child see the world from another youngster's perspective.

If the camping trip is going well, be sure to head home a little early; it prevents a last-minute meltdown. It's always better to end early on a positive note than to end with sore feet, a lot of whining, and discouraged hikers.

## . . . AND CAMPING WITH DOGS

I love camping with my dog as long as she doesn't bark at strange noises in the middle of the night. Use these basic guidelines when taking your hound into the wild.

- Leash a dog to prevent it from chasing wildlife and other campground users.
- Also leash a dog to keep it from drinking out of streams and other water sources. Harmful bacteria, such as giardia, are a threat to dogs as well as humans. Always pack water for your dog.
- Further, leash a dog to keep it from getting lost and possibly attacked by wild animals. Few

things are worse than having to take a dog to the vet on a weekend with porcupine quills lodged in its sinuses.

- Make sure that all of your dog's vaccinations and medications are current, including rabies, bordetella, and heartworm. If you're planning to camp in an area with Lyme disease, ask your vet about vaccinations.
- After camping, carefully check Fido for ticks and burrs. Prepare for accidents, and keep antibiotic cream and self-sticking bandage tape in your first-aid kid.
- It's essential to pack out dog poop rather than leave it at the campsite. Dog waste is not the same as that of other animals, even that of coyotes or wolves. It's dangerous to the environment, especially near water sources, and it makes a bad impression on the campers who use the site after you.

# EASTERN **COLORADO**

# 1
# JACKSON LAKE
# STATE PARK
# CAMPGROUND

**J**ACKSON **L**AKE **IS RANKED ONE OF** the top 15 park beaches by Reserve America. A large, warm-water reservoir, Jackson Lake is an important feature of the northeastern Colorado high plains landscape. Local farmers depend on its water to irrigate their lands. But before these waters grace the fields, they provide scenic recreational opportunities to all who are lucky enough to come this way. The Rocky Mountains will always be a draw, but this relaxing state park should not be overlooked. Campers can stay overnight in a slew of shoreline campsites while boating, sailing, swimming, and fishing on the 2,700-acre lake. A walk-in tent camping area and lakeside beaches make this oasis even more appealing.

> *Enjoy shoreline camping on this high-plains reservoir.*

Several campgrounds border the impoundment along the west shore. The Lakeside Campground has wide-open, sun-whipped campsites farther from the lake, but nearer to the water, cottonwoods shade the preferred lakeside sites. A camper's services building and shadier campsites are closer to the lake. Then a set of walk-in tent sites stretches along the shoreline. These are the best sites in the park for tent campers. A beach swimming area is near these walk-in tent sites.

The Cove Campground is more open. It has electrical hookups and caters more to RVs. The campsite picnic tables are shaded with interesting shelters that look like the shell of a turtle turned sideways. There is access to the swim beach here as well. The Pelican Campground also has four walk-in tent sites a slight distance from the shore and some shady shoreline drive-up campsites. Many of the others are more exposed to the elements. Boaters will want to take advantage of the quick access to the Shoreline Marina and boat ramp just north of the Pelican Campground.

The next campground, Sandpiper, lies on an open slope with numerous planted trees. The height of the hill allows for a great view of the lake, but at the expense

## RATINGS

**Beauty:** ✩ ✩ ✩
**Privacy:** ✩ ✩ ✩
**Spaciousness:** ✩ ✩ ✩ ✩ ✩
**Quiet:** ✩ ✩ ✩
**Security:** ✩ ✩ ✩ ✩ ✩
**Cleanliness:** ✩ ✩ ✩ ✩ ✩

# KEY INFORMATION

**ADDRESS:** Jackson Lake S. P.
26363 CR 3
Orchard, CO 80649

**OPERATED BY:** Colorado State
Parks

**INFORMATION:** (970) 645-2551;
parks.state.co.us

**OPEN:** All year

**SITES:** 262

**EACH SITE:** Picnic table, fire
ring

**ASSIGNMENT:** Reserve up to 72
hours prior to ar-
rival (For Friday
night arrival, reser-
vations need to be
made by Tuesday.)

**REGISTRATION:** (800) 678-CAMP
(2267) or (303) 470-
1144 in Denver, at
entrance station
or park office, or
online at colorado
stateparks.reserve
america.com, or by
a direct link on the
park's website

**FACILITIES:** Hot showers, flush
and vault toilets,
laundry facilities,
phone, electricity,
marina

**PARKING:** At campsites or
walk-in tent camp-
ers parking area

**FEE:** $7 Parks Pass plus
$16 per night; an
additional $10
fee added to each
Internet or phone
reservation

**ELEVATION:** 4,440 feet

**RESTRICTIONS:** *Pets:* On leash only
*Fires:* In fire grates
only
*Alcohol:* 3.2% beer
only
*Vehicles:* None
*Other:* 14-day stay
limit in a 30-day
period; quiet hours
observed 10 p.m.–
6 a.m.; camping per-
mits expire at noon

of shade and privacy. A camper's services building and electrical hookups are located here. Fox Hills is on a wide slope that offers views of the prairie and lake, which is fairly distant. There are many trees here. The final campground on the west shore, Northview, is on an open slope but has electrical hookups and shade shelters for the campsite picnic tables. These last three camp-grounds should be your last choice.

There is one small campground, Dunes, on the south shore of Jackson Lake. This campground abuts some wooded dunes that separate you from the lake, but the water is just a short climb over the dunes. The campground has picnic shelters, and also Russian olive and cottonwood trees for shade. These are popular sites, and the small size of this campground makes for a quiet camping experience.

Water sports dominate the activities at Jackson Lake. Jet skiing, power boating, and waterskiing are enjoyed during summer months. The Shoreline Marina has limited supplies and most anything a boater might need, including boats themselves, from jet skis to pon-toon barges. The west and south shores are designated as wakeless areas. In these areas are two lakeside beaches where swimmers cool off in the waters and sunbathers soak up some rays on the sand.

Bank fishing is popular in the Dike Fishing Area, where boats are prohibited. Both warm- and cold-water species inhabit the reservoir. Trout, walleye, wiper, perch, and crappie are angled for from the Dike Fishing Area and throughout the lake on boats. Anglers who go ice fishing on Jackson Lake increase each winter.

Landlubbers will be seen bicycling on the park roads. Campers can enjoy interpretive programs on summer weekends. You may learn about Jackson Lake's wildlife, especially the wealth of waterfowl. Whether on land or water, you will come away from this pride of the prairie with a new perspective on Colorado. You'll see why novelist James Michener referred to the lake as "an oasis of the plains."

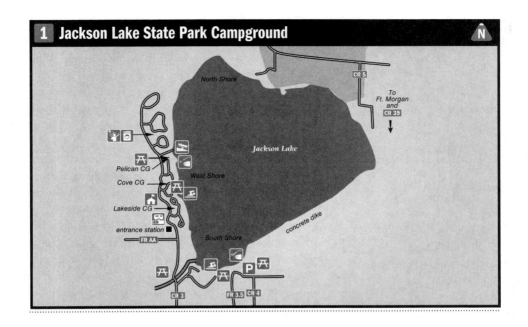

North Shore

CR 5

To
Ft. Morgan
and
CR 39

Jackson Lake

Pelican CG

West Shore

Cove CG

Lakeside CG

entrance station

FR AA

South Shore

concrete dike

CR 3

FR 3.5  CR 4

P

## GETTING THERE

From Fort Morgan, head
west on I-76 for 14 miles to
Exit 66 and CO 39. Head
north on CO 39 and follow it
for 7.3 miles to CR Y5.
Turn left on CR Y5 and
follow it 2.5 miles to
Jackson Lake State Park.

## GPS COORDINATES

**LATITUDE** N 40° 22' 50.1"
**LONGITUDE** W 104° 5' 24"

# 2
# JOHN MARTIN RESERVOIR STATE PARK:
## LAKE HASTY CAMPGROUND

> *Explore southeast Colorado and enjoy vast lake vistas.*

**J**OHN **M**ARTIN **R**ESERVOIR **S**TATE **P**ARK **HOUSES** a large lake, located 17 miles east of Las Animas. It is one of the largest reservoirs in Colorado. Many consider the park a bird-watcher's paradise. More than 400 species have been documented in the area. America's majestic bald eagle roosts here in winter. Threatened and endangered species such as the piping plover and the least tern make their home in the park for several months each year.

This remote camping experience will keep you busy with activities. This is especially true if you've never ventured into southeastern Colorado or the Lower Arkansas River Valley. The park service refers to John Martin as a "sapphire on the plains . . . a peaceful paradise." The reservoir provides under-crowded recreation: boating, waterskiing, wind water sports, fishing, and more. The mild southeastern weather provides for many sunny days all year long.

The dam that created John Martin Reservoir was built in the early 1940s as an irrigation and flood control project. Colorado State Parks took over management of the Lake Hasty area below the dam, the surface of the reservoir, and a portion of the north shore in October 2001 through a lease agreement with the U.S. Army Corps of Engineers.

Petroglyphs in the area suggest that Native Americans camped and lived here. Zebulon Pike, Kit Carson, and many other explorers and Colorado pioneers found their way into the valley. Traders and settlers traveled through the area while on the mountain route of the Santa Fe Trail. Remnants of the historic trail remain on the north shore of the park. The 4.5-mile Red Shin hiking trail begins below the dam and circles the Lake Hasty area through prairie and wetland environments. The trail then proceeds to the Santa Fe Trail market on the north shore.

## RATINGS

Beauty: ☆ ☆ ☆ ☆
Privacy: ☆ ☆ ☆
Spaciousness: ☆ ☆ ☆ ☆
Quiet: ☆ ☆ ☆
Security: ☆ ☆ ☆ ☆
Cleanliness: ☆ ☆ ☆ ☆

A total of 213 campsites in this area accommodate everything from RVs to trailers to tents. There are plenty of RV sites here, but there is enough variety of tent camping to keep you away from the large groups. The Lake Hasty Campground is located below the dam and provides plenty of shade from a canopy of mature trees. The 109 campsites have electrical hookups and modern facilities, including centrally located water hydrants, coin-operated showers, laundry facilities, and flush toilets. In winter, 51 sites remain open.

At Lake Hasty, sites 30–38 sit the closest to the shore. Site 30, a full hookup, and Site 31, a 40-foot electric, are directly across from the comfort station, showers, and laundry facilities. Site 32, a 40-foot electric, is across from the Dumpster. If you want to stay shore bound, your best bet is to snag 40-foot electric spots 33–38. Sites 10, 11, 13, 15, 18, 20, 22, 24, and 26 are 40-foot electric spots at the base of the dam and offer the privacy of an outside loop. All other sites are in a busy village of inside loops and turns within the campground.

The Lake Hasty area has parking spaces and campsites that are accessible for people of all abilities. Sites 59HA and 60HA are ADA-accessible, 40-foot electrical camping spots close to the comfort station, showers, and laundry facilities. An accessible fishing pier and picnic area are available on the west shoreline of Lake Hasty. Restrooms, showers, picnic tables, drinking fountains, and grills accommodate everyone.

The Point Campground is located on the north shore; it sits on a ridge overlooking John Martin Reservoir. No electricity, water, or shade is available, but the views of the landscape are exceptional. Vault toilets are available. The Point is closed during the winter. Campsites 201–304 are considered 40-foot non-electrical basic. These 104 sites are located at the Point and are some of the best options for tent campers. Sites 271–275, 295, and 296 sit on two outside loops and offer fantastic views. Sites 214, 215, 231, and 232 are on busier loops, but they are spread apart and have the advantage of being on the outside edges.

Fishing and water sports dominate recreation at John Martin Reservoir. Hand-propelled craft, sailboats, and boats with electric motors are permitted on Lake

| | |
|---|---|
| **ADDRESS:** | John Martin S. P. 30703 CR 24 Hasty, CO 81044 |
| **OPERATED BY:** | Colorado State Parks |
| **INFORMATION:** | (719) 829-1801; parks.state.co.us |
| **OPEN:** | All year |
| **SITES:** | 109 (51 sites open in winter) |
| **EACH SITE HAS:** | Picnic table, fire ring, electric hookups |
| **ASSIGNMENT:** | Campsites must be reserved |
| **REGISTRATION:** | (800) 678-CAMP (2267) or (303) 470-1144 in Denver, at entrance station or park office, or online at colorado stateparks.reserve america.com, or by a direct link on the park's website |
| **FACILITIES:** | Hot showers, flush and vault toilets, laundry facilities, phone, electricity, swimming beach, playground |
| **PARKING:** | At campsite |
| **FEE:** | $7 Parks Pass plus $16 per night; additional $10 fee added to each Internet or phone reservation |
| **ELEVATION:** | 3,851 feet |
| **RESTRICTIONS:** | *Pets:* On leash only *Fires:* In fire grates only *Alcohol:* 3.2% beer only *Vehicles:* One vehicle per campsite unless space permits *Other:* 14-day stay limit in a 45-day period |

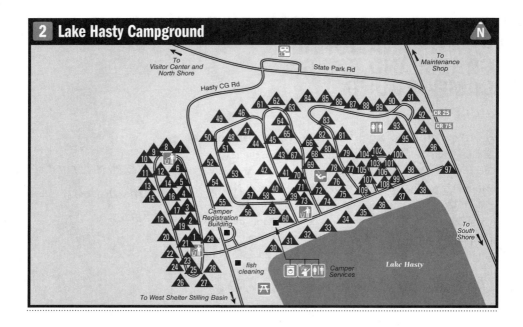

## GETTING THERE

From Las Animas, take CO 50 east for 17 miles to Hasty. From Hasty, head south on CR 24 for 2 miles. The park visitor center will be on the right.

## GPS COORDINATES

**LATITUDE** N 38° 04' 29"
**LONGITUDE** W 102° 55' 50"

Hasty. John Martin Reservoir is open to all types of boating. Swimming is designated at the swim beach at Lake Hasty below the dam. Fishing is permitted, if you have a valid fishing license, anywhere in the park, except from the boat docks and all areas closed to public access. The most common species caught at John Martin include walleye, saugeye, bass, crappies, muskie, wiper, catfish, perch, and bluegill. Lake Hasty is stocked in spring and fall with rainbow trout and cutthroat trout, which can be fished from the shore around the lake.

# 3
# PAWNEE NATIONAL GRASSLAND FAMILY CAMPGROUND

**I**F THE COLORADO MOUNTAINS ARE WHAT make the state famous, then the Colorado prairies are the lesser-known better half. And the humble prairie folk are okay with that. The uninterrupted vistas and heritage of Northeastern Colorado comprise an open book of nature with its own distinct and fragile beauty. Less populated and less trampled by tourists, this area is prime for discovery. Tent campgrounds are extremely limited east of I-25, the main interstate artery that loosely splits the state in half and serves as a vein to the Colorado Front Range. So, we are pleased to point you in the direction of Pawnee National Grassland and the Crow Valley Recreation Area.

*Head east for a high-plains pioneer experience.*

Traveling across the Pawnee Pioneer Trail Scenic and Historic Byway, you may imagine how this short grass prairie was viewed by Native Americans, frontier men and women, early cattle ranchers, homesteaders, and those who faced the Dust Bowl and Great Depression of the 1930s. After the failure of many farms during this last timeframe, the US government purchased land from bankrupt farmers and instituted methods to restore the land and vegetation damaged by years of drought, plowing, wind, and water; thus creating the Pawnee National Grassland. Today, the Pawnee National Grassland covers almost 200,000 acres mixed with private land and is an internationally known birding area. Hiking, camping, picnicking, mountain biking, and sight-seeing are also popular recreational activities.

The campground is just past the entrance to the Crow Valley Recreation Area, which is only a quarter mile off CR 77. When you enter, pass by group picnicking and camping sites and the turnoff for the education site. Crow Valley Campground sits along Crow Creek, and the entrance is right next to the Birdwalk Trailhead. A grove of elm and cottonwood trees provides a unique respite in an otherwise open prairie. There are ten individual sites and they begin in a counterclockwise

## RATINGS

Beauty: ✩ ✩ ✩ ✩
Privacy: ✩ ✩ ✩ ✩
Spaciousness: ✩ ✩ ✩
Quiet: ✩ ✩ ✩ ✩
Security: ✩ ✩ ✩
Cleanliness: ✩ ✩ ✩

## KEY INFORMATION

**ADDRESS:** Pawnee National Grassland
44741 WCR 77
Briggsdale, CO
80611

**OPERATED BY:** USDA Forest Service, Arapaho and Roosevelt National Forests, Pawnee National Grassland

**INFORMATION:** (970) 346-5000, www.fs.fed.us/arnf

**OPEN:** April–September

**SITES:** 10

**EACH SITE:** Picnic table, fire pit

**ASSIGNMENT:** Reserve online at recreation.gov or call (877) 444-6777

**REGISTRATION:** On site

**FACILITIES:** Water, vault toilets, horseshoe pits, volleyball court, baseball field, and farm museum

**PARKING:** At campsite

**FEE:** $10 per day for a single unit, $14 per day for a double unit; reservations are from 2 p.m. day one to 2 p.m. the last day of your stay

**ELEVATION:** 4,856 feet

**RESTRICTIONS:** *Pets:* On leash
*Fires:* In designated fire pits
*Alcohol:* Allowed
*Vehicles:* 35 feet
*Other:* 14-day stay limit; single units hold 5 people, double units hold 10 people

layout around a perfect circle. All campsites meet ADA requirements for handicap accessibility. (There are also two accessible trails in the campground.) One double unit is available for those with special needs, and the rangers ask that you leave this unit open until all other spaces are filled. Sites 1, 2, and 3 are single campsites on the outer edge of the circle. Following them are sites 4, 5, and 6, which are the three double campsites. Sites 7, 8, 9, and 10 are closer to Crow Creek and sit on the western edge of the circle. Site 9 is the only site in the middle of the circle.

May and June are the best months to visit because the bird migration is in full swing, wildflowers are in bloom, and it is much cooler than the blazing July and August months. Even during the cooler months, finding a shady campsite among the ten is paramount. Large cottonwood trees shade the sites that ring the outer fringe of the campground. From these sites, short trails lead through the Crow Valley cottonwood groves and river thickets that attract birds and birders in large numbers. July and August are not only hot, but the mosquitoes swarm. If you come during these hot months be prepared.

Pawnee National Grassland offers hiking opportunities directly from the campground and within the prairie. The Pawnee Buttes are 30 miles northeast of the Crow Valley Recreation Area. The Buttes rise 300 feet above the surrounding prairie and are the result of erosion of uplifted sedimentary beds deposited by ancient seas. The trail is open all year and is an easy 1.5-mile hike to the base of the western Pawnee Butte.

Pawnee National Grassland supports many bird species, especially during migration. The Colorado state bird, the lark bunting, is very common in the prairie in the spring and summer. A pamphlet, describing a self-guided motor vehicle bird tour of the west side of the Pawnee National Grassland, is available in Crow Valley. A brochure titled "Birding on the Pawnee by Automobile or Mountain Bike" is even available for mountain bikers. The history of the area is represented by many cemeteries, small museums, and preserved homesteads. Artifacts, arrowheads, fossils, and antique barnwood are easy to spot, but you must leave these items untouched.

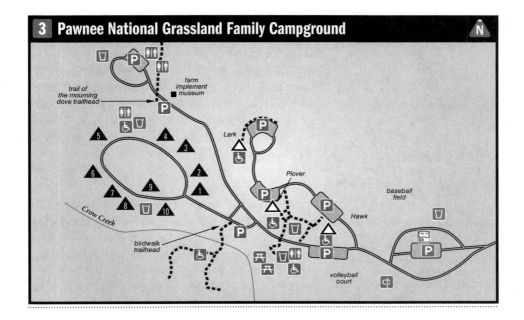

Keep this campground at the top of your flatland list. It is an eye-opening experience to witness the magic of Colorado from the solitude of its open spaces. The mountain views are much different here than anywhere else in the state, with distant views of the snow-capped peaks. Large, fluffy clouds turn into dark thunderheads in a snap, and lightning illuminates the beasts, creating quite a show. This, along with the promise of no crowds and your pick of campsites, should seal the deal.

## GETTING THERE

From the intersection of I-25 and CO 14, take CO 14 east 37 miles to Weld County Road CR 77. Take CR 77 a quarter mile to the campground.

## GPS COORDINATES

**LATITUDE** N 40 °38' 45"
**LONGITUDE** W 104° 20' 14"

# 4
# SOUTH REPUBLICAN STATE WILDLIFE AREA CAMPGROUND

> *South Republican is your prairie getaway in northeastern Colorado.*

**S**OUTH REPUBLICAN IS THE MOST EASTERLY campground in this entire guidebook. Located in a wide valley of the South Fork of the Republican River near the Kansas border, this 1,900-acre reservoir was originally built by the U.S. Bureau of Reclamation in the 1950s. The state of Colorado transformed it into a state park in the 1970s. Now, the former Bonny Lake State Park is part of the South Republican State Wildlife Area. The merging of the former state park and the South Republican State Wildlife Area creates a 13,000-acre management unit that offers deer, turkey, waterfowl, and small game hunting.

Now you can enjoy this surprisingly scenic slice of the prairie "almost" all by yourself. Until the future of the former state park is finalized, the fate of the other large campgrounds and facilities remains in limbo. The East Beach is the best in tent camping among the good group of campgrounds that circled the lake. If you are coming from out of state, stop here on your way to or from the mountains. You will realize that Colorado really is beautiful not only in the high country, but in the prairie as well.

Some campgrounds and other visitor services are closed, but the good news is that the East Beach Campground will remain open with primitive camping—perfect for tent campers . . . no water or electricity . . . no RVs. Starting on the northwest side of Bonny Lake is the former Foster Grove Campground. The former North Cove is on a small arm of the lake. The campground is smaller but was more popular than Foster Grove. On the southern shore of Bonny Lake near the main body of park development is the former Wagon Wheel Campground. Its many RV-like amenities, including laundry facilities, a dump station, and electricity, are now closed.

The East Beach Campground is at the southeastern corner of the reservoir near the dam. Drive in and pass

## RATINGS

Beauty: ✿ ✿ ✿ ✿
Privacy: ✿ ✿ ✿ ✿
Spaciousness: ✿ ✿ ✿
Quiet: ✿ ✿ ✿ ✿
Security: ✿ ✿ ✿ ✿
Cleanliness: ✿ ✿ ✿ ✿ ✿

three sunny campsites near the lake—they are screened from a view of the beach area by a line of cottonwoods. Under this line of cottonwoods are the park's best campsites. This is a row of ten walk-in tent sites, which are by the lake under the trees and have a view of the beautiful waters. Try to get these campsites. Farther on are 20 more campsites exposed to the extremes of the prairie—mainly open exposure, high winds, and blazing sunshine. Thankfully, they do have shade shelters. The lake dam stands tall to your right.

Bonny Lake is a reservoir, and state engineers drain the reservoir periodically, releasing water to Kansas and Nebraska to comply with the Republican River Compact, which divides the water between the three states. This process also marks the beginning of the seasonal waterfowl resting period and the end of fishing at Bonny Lake. Hale Ponds offers warm-water fishing. Call ahead or check the website for the latest fishing report.

The view of the waters and the prairie from the dam is a vivid delight. Bonny Lake and her new alias are not just for summer. Wildlife viewing is a year-round pastime here, and there is more wildlife here than at many other plains reservoirs and river bottoms. Birdlife is particularly abundant. Hunting is allowed in season. No matter what time of year you visit, you will be pleasantly surprised at this old, new, growing, and transitioning area.

## KEY INFORMATION

**ADDRESS:** Brush Area Office—DOW
122 E Edison St.
Brush, CO 80723

**OPERATED BY:** Colorado Division of Wildlife

**INFORMATION:** (970) 354-7317 or (970) 842-6300; wildlife.state.co.us/landwater/state wildlifeareas; Sheriff's Office, Yuma, (970) 332-4805

**OPEN:** All year

**SITES:** 10 walk-in tent sites

**EACH SITE:** Picnic table and stand-up grill

**ASSIGNMENT:** First come, first served

**REGISTRATION:** Not needed

**FACILITIES:** Restrooms and picnic shelters

**PARKING:** At walk-in tent campers parking area

**FEE:** None

**ELEVATION:** 3,700 feet

**RESTRICTIONS:** *Pets:* Not allowed
*Fires:* In fire grates only
*Alcohol:* Allowed
*Vehicles:* Designated roads only
*Other:* 14-day stay limit in 45-day period; obey CDOW rules and regulations; be aware of hunters in season; respect private property

**4 South Republican State Wildlife Area**

## GETTING THERE

From I-70 in Burlington, drive north on US 385 for 23 miles to CR 2. Turn right on CR 2 and follow it 1.5 miles to the former Bonny Lake State Park.

## GPS COORDINATES

**LATITUDE** N 39° 36' 30.8"
**LONGITUDE** W 102° 11' 16"

NORTH CENTRAL **COLORADO**

# 5 BROWNS PARK CAMPGROUND

**T**HE LOWER **L**ARAMIE **R**IVER **VALLEY** HAS a big-country-lonesome feel to it. There aren't too many folks around here, mainly just ranchers. Browns Park is tucked away in some woods on a side creek that feeds into the Laramie. If you want to get away from the people who are trying to get away from it all, come here. This pretty little campground is adjacent to the woods and lakes of the Rawah Wilderness, which covers a stretch of the Medicine Bow Mountains. You can hike and fish here, or just take it easy. Browns Park is great for relaxation. Summer afternoons are as slow as molasses.

After passing the busy campgrounds of the Poudre Canyon and overcrowded Chambers Lake, you'll feel grateful for the peace and quiet here in the Laramie Valley.

A couple of sites lie in the lodgepole and aspen woods to your right, then the main campground drive splits off to the right and you enter the outer loop. (There used to be one more split off to the right, but the beavers took care of that.) The outer loop turns away from Jinks Creek and runs alongside a slight slope.

The campsites on the outside of the loop are higher than the road, but have been graded and host tent pads for a level night of rest. The inner loop campsites lie in a mixed wood with a very grassy understory augmented by small conifers. Move away from the hill and pass the inner loop. These campsites are more open, but all are spread far apart, so privacy can be had by every camper. The inner loop splits Browns Park in half, but the roads are spread far enough apart that you won't be bothered by your fellow campers when they drive past. The county road leading in to Browns Park gets less traffic than some campgrounds I've seen.

Complete your loop back to the campground entrance and the vault toilets. Browns Park has no water—I recommend bringing it with you.

> *Browns Park abuts the old-growth forests and alpine lakes of the Rawah Wilderness near the Wyoming border.*

## RATINGS

**Beauty:** ☆ ☆ ☆ ☆
**Privacy:** ☆ ☆ ☆
**Spaciousness:** ☆ ☆ ☆ ☆
**Quiet:** ☆ ☆ ☆ ☆
**Security:** ☆ ☆ ☆
**Cleanliness:** ☆ ☆ ☆

# KEY INFORMATION

**ADDRESS:** Browns Park Campground Canyon Lakes Ranger District 2150 Centre Ave., Builing E Fort Collins, CO 80526

**OPERATED BY:** USDA Forest Service, Arapaho and Roosevelt National Forests, Pawnee National Grassland

**INFORMATION:** (970) 295-6700; www.fs.fed.us

**OPEN:** May–September

**SITES:** 28

**EACH SITE:** Tent pad, picnic table, fire grate, stand-up grill

**ASSIGNMENT:** First come, first served; no reservations

**REGISTRATION:** Self-registration on site

**FACILITIES:** Vault toilet (no water)

**PARKING:** At campsites only

**FEE:** $11 per night

**ELEVATION:** 8,400 feet

**RESTRICTIONS:** *Pets:* On leash only *Fires:* In fire grates only *Alcohol:* At campsites only *Vehicles:* 30 feet *Other:* 14-day stay limit

This campground has low usage. I met a man on my visit who had been coming to Browns Park for ten years and had only seen the campground full once. He and his wife were the only campers there on the day I met him. Weekdays can be desolate, which is great for those who love solitude. Summer weekends can be half to two-thirds full, except when the campground fills up for major holidays.

For a nearby natural experience, check out the beaver pond and see if you find any of nature's architects plotting to flood the rest of the campground. Two hiking trails leave from the trailhead adjacent to Browns Park into the Rawah Wilderness, which is far enough from the metropolitan areas to receive little use also.

The McIntyre Trail traces McIntyre Creek to Houseman Park, and then turns left to another meadow where beavers have again been busy flooding the trail. These upper beaver ponds offer excellent trout fishing. The Link Trail climbs through a lodgepole forest to a former burned area, where views of the Laramie River valley stretch into Wyoming. You can also see the Poudre Canyon below.

If you want to access the high lakes of the Medicine Bows, take the Rawah Trail, which starts in the Laramie River valley south of Browns Park (you pass this trailhead on the way in). The Rawah Trail crosses several different environments. Leave the valley grasslands, wind your way from lodgepole to spruce-fir forest to tundra above the tree line, where there are many bodies of water collectively dubbed the Rawah Lakes.

No matter what you do, bring some friends with you to Browns Park and the Medicine Bows because there might not be too many other people out here, especially during the week. Also, bring all the supplies you may need because the nearest store is not really near at all, though there is a guest ranch nearby down Larimer CR 103.

## GETTING THERE

From Fort Collins drive north on US 287 for 11 miles to CO 14. Turn left on CO 14 and follow it for 49 miles west to CR 103 (Laramie River Road). Turn right on CR 103 and follow it for 15 miles. At a T-intersection turn left on CR 80C and travel approximately 3 miles to Browns Park Campground.

## GPS COORDINATES

| | |
|---|---|
| LATITUDE | N 40° 47' 49.7" |
| LONGITUDE | W 105° 55' 37" |

# 6
# BUFFALO CAMPGROUND

*Buffalo is a quick getaway for metro Denver–area mountain bikers, hikers, and families.*

**S**O MANY OF THE BEST NATIONAL-FOREST campgrounds are high in the Rockies, where the weather and roads can be rough. Buffalo Campground, at 7,400 feet, is high enough to escape the heat of the lowlands, but not so high that you'll be dressing for winter in July. A network of trails, including the Colorado Trail, winds through the immediate area of ponderosa pines and strange rock formations that burst forth from the needle-carpeted forest floor. This haven in the Pike National Forest is only 70 miles from the metropolitan Denver area.

Buffalo is situated in a stand of mature ponderosa pine on a gentle slope. Flowers, grasses, and juniper ground cover spread over the open, parklike forest floor. An ideal mix of sun and shade makes its way through the evergreens onto the very large campsites. The largest of tents will have no problem fitting on the leveled areas at each campsite. But this openness cuts down on camper privacy.

Pass the fee station and begin climbing up the hillside. Pass an inner loop that splits off to your left and has seven campsites that are more open than most because they border a small clearing in the center of the main loop. Most of the campsites are on the outside of the main loop and extend far back from the road. The higher you are on the loop, the better you can see a stone outcrop across the way where rock climbers go to work.

A campground host is stationed on the loop to quell any late-night parties or direct you to the many recreational opportunities in the area. The campground was recently refurbished, and its vault toilets have been replaced. The three water spigots are very reliable.

You can reserve a site here, but Buffalo rarely fills, barring major summer holidays. Weekends usually see a mix of families and youthful active folks, the vast majority of whom are tent campers. Buffalo is quiet during the

## RATINGS

Beauty: ✿ ✿ ✿ ✿
Privacy: ✿ ✿
Spaciousness: ✿ ✿ ✿ ✿ ✿
Quiet: ✿ ✿ ✿
Security: ✿ ✿ ✿ ✿
Cleanliness: ✿ ✿ ✿

week; you can be assured of a campsite. No matter when you come, there is plenty to enjoy in the surrounding Pike National Forest.

As mentioned, rock climbers scale the formation across from the campground. Mountain bikers are seen everywhere, riding the trails that wind through the Buffalo Recreation Area and beyond. A favorite ride is the Colorado Trail. Keep going up the hill from the campground and you will intersect the trail. You can turn left out of the campground on the Colorado Trail and bike to CO 126, then return via FS 550. Trail 722 makes a loop off the Colorado Trail south. Just off FS 550, there is another loop that heads toward Miller Gulch. Make up your own loop in the trails that twist and turn amid the pines and pillars of stone.

Buffalo Creek, flowing just below the campground, offers trout fishing and more mountain biking along FS 543, which parallels Buffalo. Still more biking trails splinter off FS 543. Wellington Lake, at the upper drainage of Buffalo Creek, is a private lake that offers boat rentals and trout fishing for a fee.

Hikers can enjoy the same trails as the mountain bikers. You can also head into the Lost Creek Wilderness, just a few miles northwest of Buffalo. From the trailhead off Wellington Lake Road, hikers can take the Colorado Trail into the wilderness high country or walk the Craig Meadows Trail into Craig Creek. Other hikes into this wilderness are also accessible from this trailhead.

In the summer there is still enough light to make the drive from Denver or Colorado Springs and be sitting at Buffalo at dusk by the campfire, where you can cook up a good supper, then retire to your tent. Next morning you can jump out of the tent and onto your favorite trail.

## KEY INFORMATION

| | |
|---|---|
| **ADDRESS:** | Buffalo Campground 28718 Redskin Creek Rd. Bailey, CO 80421 |
| **OPERATED BY:** | USDA Forest Service, Pike and San Isabel National Forests, Cimarron and Comanche National Grasslands |
| **INFORMATION:** | (303) 275-5610; www.fs.fed.us |
| **OPEN:** | Mid-May–Labor Day |
| **SITES:** | 41 |
| **EACH SITE:** | Picnic table, fire ring, tent pad |
| **ASSIGNMENT:** | By reservation |
| **REGISTRATION:** | Call (877) 444-6777 or visit reserveusa.com |
| **FACILITIES:** | Water spigot, vault toilet |
| **PARKING:** | At campsites only |
| **FEE:** | $14 per night, with additional $9 fee added to each Internet or phone reservation |
| **ELEVATION:** | 7,400 feet |
| **RESTRICTIONS:** | *Pets:* On leash only *Fires:* In fire rings only *Alcohol:* At campsites only *Vehicles:* 22 feet *Other:* 14-day stay limit |

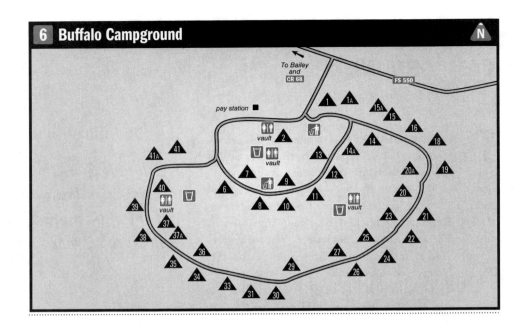

## GETTING THERE

From US 285 in Bailey, head southeast on CR 68 (it turns into FS 543) for 8 miles to FS 550. Turn left on FS 550 (Redskin Creek Road) and follow it 4 miles to Buffalo (not Buffalo Springs) Campground, which will be on your right.

## GPS COORDINATES

**LATITUDE** N 39° 20' 32.9"
**LONGITUDE** W 105° 20' 8.3"

# 7
# THE CRAGS CAMPGROUND

*Gould*

**T**HE **CRAGS IS AN APPROPRIATE NAME** for this campground. It is balanced on the steep slopes of the Never Summer Mountains. The treeless, granite precipices are not far above you and your vista of Diamond Peaks. The actual Nokhu Crags are behind you and out of sight from the campground. The camping season is short, and nights are always cool here. So reserve a piece of your valuable time in July or August and see what the Colorado State Forest has to offer.

This forest actually abuts Rocky Mountain National Park, so that ought to give you an idea of the level of scenery here. North Park, the vast expanse of meadowland in Jackson County, is known as the moose capital of Colorado. Plan to see a few of those large critters and a few more animals if you explore the trails of Colorado State Forest.

After you drive that dizzying last mile to The Crags, take a deep breath and enter the campground. The setting is a high-country forest of subalpine fir and Engelmann spruce growing densely on steep slopes. Fear not, for the campsites have been leveled, though you may have to go up or down a bit to reach the camp from your car.

Don't drive too fast through the loop or you'll miss some of the campsites, which are set back in the woods. A few sites have pull-through areas for your vehicle, but don't expect to see any big rigs up here. That road discourages them, but any passenger car smaller than a moving truck can make the drive.

Enter a sunny area where you will see tree stumps left over from the days when this area was logged. Campsites here have a clear view of the severe lands above them. The loop reenters the woods, and the more heavily wooded campsites begin. The last three sites are very isolated and offer the most solitude. Back at the beginning of the loop are vault toilets for each gender;

*Colorado State Forest is rich in wildlife and is one of the state's best places to see moose.*

## RATINGS

Beauty: ✿ ✿ ✿
Privacy: ✿ ✿ ✿ ✿
Spaciousness: ✿ ✿ ✿
Quiet: ✿ ✿ ✿ ✿
Security: ✿ ✿ ✿
Cleanliness: ✿ ✿ ✿

# KEY INFORMATION

the hand-pump well is to your left in the woods a bit. The water here is very cold.

Weekdays rarely find the campground filled. However, on later summer weekends, it will be alive with families and young couples, along with a few from the older generation who haven't converted to the dreaded RV. But this hidden jewel of a park is not nearly as busy as other Front Range parks.

The Crags is close to some of the 71,000-acre Colorado State Forest's best hiking. Just up the road is the trail to Lake Agnes. It is less than a mile from the trailhead to the lake, which is banked against the Nokhu Crags. A path makes a loop around the lake. American Lakes are accessible by a 5-mile hike and offer views of the Medicine Bow Mountains. Make the one-way walk to Cameron Pass and have a shuttle car pick you up. You might see mountain lions, elk, mule deer, coyotes, and bears.

Ruby Jewel Lake is only a 1.5-mile trek. Kelly Lake and Clear Lake are other destination hikes in the park. If you fish these waters, remember that only artificial lures and flies are allowed. State regulations apply in park streams and in North Michigan Reservoir and Ranger Lakes.

Check out the visitor center with the unique barbed-wire moose outside and the stuffed moose inside. There are also informative displays on the park's wildlife that kids will really love.

In 1995, the Colorado Senate declared North Park the Moose Capital of Colorado. Moose were introduced into North Park in the late 1970s and have been thriving here ever since. Try to observe moose in the early morning and late evening in the willow thickets along area creeks. You should also take the auto tour of the Arapaho National Wildlife Refuge in the heart of North Park. Get directions at the visitor center.

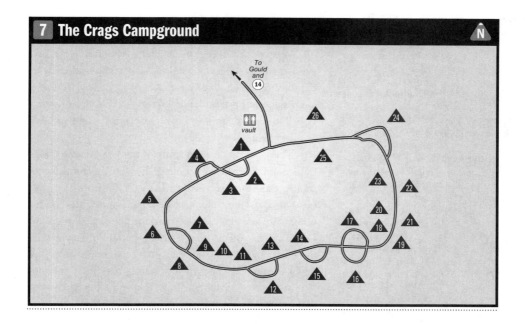

## GETTING THERE

From Gould, drive north on CO 14 for 7 miles to FS 170. There will be a sign for Lake Agnes. Turn right on FS 170 and follow it for 0.5 mile to the first intersection. Turn right on FS 172 and climb steeply for 1 mile, turning left at the next intersection. Continue to The Crags Campground.

## GPS COORDINATES

| | |
|---|---|
| LATITUDE | N 40° 29' 19.3" |
| LONGITUDE | W 105° 54' 14" |

# 8
# ELBERT CREEK CAMPGROUND

*You can walk from your tent and hike up Mount Elbert, Colorado's highest peak at 14,433 feet.*

**A**CTIVE CAMPERS COME TO **E**LBERT **C**REEK, and it seems that they are not around enough to really take in the atmosphere of the campground. Elbert Creek has an agreeable location, high in the mountains along a resonant stream, where you really get a sense of being away from it all. But campers here seem to think they are near it all, at least those exercise-oriented pastimes that active campers like. Hiking is the main exercise; Mount Elbert and the Mount Massive Wilderness are just a walk away from the campground.

There are lakes and streams nearby for fishing. Mountain bikers like to pedal up to Mount Champion Mill and the Colorado Trail—the backbone of the state's trail system. Somehow, campers find time to eat, sleep, and rest a little before going at it again the next day.

Elbert Creek is a small campground laid out underneath a lodgepole-pine forest in a flat along Halfmoon Creek. Enter the campground and the road splits into two drives running parallel to Halfmoon Creek that have vehicle turnarounds at their ends. This avails more streamside campsites. The forest is virtually devoid of ground cover, save for a few small saplings and rocks. However, the brush thickens alongside Halfmoon Creek, which flows loud and clear below the campground.

The right-hand drive has nine campsites. Many of these sites are spread far back in the woods. Four of the campsites are streamside and offer solitude. The left-hand drive has eight campsites that are very large, but three of them are a little close to the forest road that runs by the campground. Avoid the last three campsites unless you want to see who is driving by.

The pump well and vault toilets are conveniently located between the two drives. Elbert Creek receives heavy weekend use from hikers, so try to get there on Friday night or early Saturday if you are a weekend warrior. Otherwise, campsites are nearly always available.

## RATINGS

Beauty: ✿ ✿ ✿ ✿
Privacy: ✿ ✿ ✿
Spaciousness: ✿ ✿ ✿ ✿ ✿
Quiet: ✿ ✿ ✿
Security: ✿ ✿ ✿
Cleanliness: ✿ ✿ ✿

Hikers love to bag peaks here in the Centennial State, and the highest point in Colorado, Mount Elbert, is very close. Elbert is the second-highest point in the lower 48 states, behind Mount Whitney in California. It is a 3.5-mile climb to the crest from the nearby trailhead. There's nothing technical about this well-marked and maintained trail, though snow may present a problem even in the early summer. You can also make a loop hike from here using the North Mount Elbert, South Mount Elbert, and Colorado Trails.

Just a short walk up the road is the Mount Massive Wilderness. Much of this wilderness is above the timber line, so bring adequate clothing for inclement weather. Mount Massive is the second-highest peak in Colorado, only 12 feet lower than Mount Elbert. You can stay at Elbert Creek and climb the two highest peaks in the state. Just beyond the Mount Elbert Trailhead, take the Colorado Trail north into the wilderness up to the Mount Massive Trail and hike to the peak. You can also climb to the North Halfmoon Lakes using Trail 1485, which starts up FS 110 a couple of miles. Farther up this same road is the Champion Mine, with its aerial tramway still intact. You can bike or drive to the Champion Mine.

The Iron Mike Mine site is a hike or bike up South Halfmoon Creek. Nearby Emerald Lake features a picnic area and offers fishing, as do all the previously mentioned creeks. Speaking of fish, you ought to check out the Leadville National Fish Hatchery. Established in 1889, it is the second-oldest federal fish hatchery in the country. Fish from here have been placed all over the Rockies, and today it still produces brook, cutthroat trout, and rainbow trout. There are trails on the hatchery grounds as well, with great views of the big mountains you came here to climb.

## KEY INFORMATION

| | |
|---|---|
| **ADDRESS:** | Elbert Creek Campground Leadville Ranger District 810 Front Street Leadville, CO 80461 |
| **OPERATED BY:** | USDA Forest Service, Pike and San Isabel National Forests, Cimarron and Comanche National Grasslands |
| **INFORMATION:** | (719) 486-0749; www.fs.fed.us |
| **OPEN:** | June–Labor Day |
| **SITES:** | 17 |
| **EACH SITE:** | Picnic table, fire grate |
| **ASSIGNMENT:** | First come, first served; no reservations |
| **REGISTRATION:** | Self-registration on site |
| **FACILITIES:** | Pump well, vault toilets, trash collection |
| **PARKING:** | At campsites only |
| **FEE:** | $13 per night |
| **ELEVATION:** | 10,100 feet |
| **RESTRICTIONS:** | *Pets:* On leash only *Fires:* In fire grates only *Alcohol:* At campsites only *Vehicles:* 16 feet *Other:* 14-day stay limit |

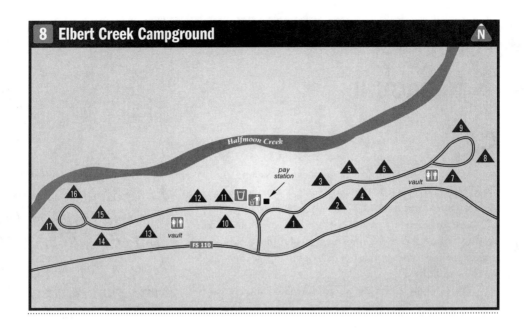

## GETTING THERE

From Leadville, head south on US 24 for 4 miles to CR 110 and the sign for the Leadville National Fish Hatchery. Turn right here and follow CR 110 for 0.7 mile to Halfmoon Creek Road. Turn left on Halfmoon Creek Road and follow it a short ways before the sharp right turn to stay on Half-moon Creek Road. Continue on Halfmoon Creek Road as it turns into FS 110. Elbert Creek Campground will be 4 miles up on your right.

## GPS COORDINATES

**LATITUDE** N 39° 9' 16.5"
**LONGITUDE** W 106° 24' 22"

# 9
# FLATIRON RESERVOIR CAMPGROUND

**M**ANY OF THE MILLIONS OF TOURISTS that arrive in Rocky Mountain National Park do so via Loveland. But, the tent campsites between Loveland and Estes Park are few and far between. Thank goodness for Flatiron Campground. Not only is it easy to get to off the main highway to the park, it is a great place to rest up before the real games begin. The place is tidy, campsites are spaced apart nicely, and the scenery is quite beautiful.

The campground is just west of Loveland and is adjacent to Larimer County Parks and Open Lands' Carter Lake, Pinewood Lake, and Ramsay-Shockey Open Space. The landscape here is semiarid with brush, small trees, red rock, and bluffs. Flatiron Reservoir itself includes 47 acres of water, plus 200 acres of public lands. This small lake is framed by Flatiron Mountain, a large, red bluff on the eastern side that towers over the water and the campground, which sits on the western edge of the water.

If you are looking for a place to rest before or after you tackle Rocky Mountain National Park, this is the place. The other Larimer County open spaces in this area also provide camping access, but Flatiron Reservoir shines above them all. The campground is approximately 10 minutes from Loveland and about 40 minutes from Estes Park. The drive up the Thompson Canyon is a long crawl, especially during the summer months when campers are practically bumper to bumper up the winding road. If you can, time your visit in the early fall and not only will it cut your drive time, you may also be able to use Flatiron Campground as a base camp for exploring Rocky Mountain National Park.

Flatiron Campground lies along Flatiron Reservoir, where boating and swimming are prohibited. Flatiron Mountain sits directly across the water, and the landscape breaks up the rest of the campground. Residential areas and the Flatiron Powerplant are adjacent to the

*Great camping east of Rocky Mountain National Park and really the only option between Loveland, a main park gateway, and Estes Park.*

## RATINGS

**Beauty:** ✩ ✩ ✩
**Privacy:** ✩ ✩ ✩
**Spaciousness:** ✩ ✩ ✩
**Quiet:** ✩ ✩ ✩
**Security:** ✩ ✩ ✩ ✩
**Cleanliness:** ✩ ✩ ✩ ✩

# KEY INFORMATION

**ADDRESS:** Flatiron Reservoir Larimer County Parks and Open Lands Department 1800 South CR 31 Loveland, CO 80537

**OPERATED BY:** Larimer County

**INFORMATION:** (970) 679-4570; larimer.org/parks

**OPEN:** All year

**SITES:** 37, plus 2 camp cabins

**EACH SITE:** Fire grate, picnic table

**ASSIGNMENT:** By reservation

**REGISTRATION:** (800) 397-7795 or larimercamping .com, or check in with camp host

**FACILITIES:** Vault toilets, water, wheelchair-accessible fishing pier, volleyball, horseshoe pit

**PARKING:** At sites or walk-in tent campers parking area

**FEE:** $15 per night, plus $7 entrance permit, plus reservation fee

**ELEVATION:** 5,470 feet

**RESTRICTIONS:** *Pets:* Leashed *Fires:* In designated grates only *Alcohol:* 3.2% beer permitted, glass prohibited *Vehicles:* 30 feet *Other:* Capacity varies by site; maximum 8 people in largest sites; no boating; 14-day stay limit; stay 100 feet away from dam; quiet hours 10 p.m.–6 a.m.

campground but are not visible from most campsites. The first nine sites are adjacent to the group day-use area, but far enough from the water to offer some privacy. The host is here, and many of the smaller RVs tend to pick these spots. Continue up the main drive, and to the right is site F10, with large trees, plenty of shade, and proximity to the water. Across the road is site F11, which looks like it gets the brunt of the traffic and wouldn't be my first pick.

Right before the main loop starts on a right spur, the main tent sites and cabins come up on the left and a good site, F12, sits to the right. I consider all of the sites at Flatiron Campground to be good for tents, but these sites have walk-in access only. The two cabins look neat, and each also has an additional tent pad. Campsites F36 and F37 are similar, shaded, and close together; F35 is higher up on an overlook, does not offer much shade, and appears to be very exposed.

Once the road spurs to the right, you enter the waterfront camping zone. Sites F13, F14, F16, F18, F20, F21, and F24 are all on the water and are very similar in that they have beautiful views, privacy, and plenty of space. Of the seven, F16 was my favorite. The sites across the road are nice but a little more exposed; F19 is a handicapped-accessible site. Continuing on is another small spur that leads to two campsites (F26 and F27) that offer good privacy. At the turn to these sites are two sites (F28 and F25) that are too close to the main county road and are not that nice. Circle back along the loop and most of the sites here are higher up and more exposed. Site F33 is off to the side and hosts four large pines; F34 is in the middle section but has some nice trees as well.

Many folks come to Flatiron Campground to trout fish, relax, or just picnic for the day. The Bison Visitor Center is close to the campground and has plenty of information on the area and tempts you with myriad recreational activities. If you feel like getting cleaned up and spending money, an outlet shopping center and a new lifestyle mall sit on the far eastern edge of Loveland near I-25.

If you really want a change of pace, there are many areas along this Colorado Front Range corridor and into Wyoming that are accessible from Flatiron Campground.

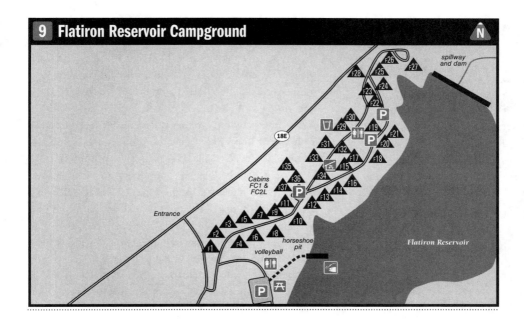

## GETTING THERE

Go north to Fort Collins (30-minute drive) and enjoy the town or the outdoor recreation close to town. Horse-tooth Reservoir, Lory State Park, and Poudre Canyon are honorable mentions. If you go south, you can sample the fun of Boulder (30-minute drive) or Denver (1-hour drive). Or, go even farther north into Wyoming (1-hour drive) and open up a whole new world of western fun.

To get to Loveland, you probably drove north on I-25. From Loveland, drive west on CO 34 to CR 29 (also known as Carter Lake Road). Turn right onto CR 18E, travel 2.6 miles, end at Flatiron Reservoir.

## GPS COORDINATES

| | |
|---|---|
| **LATITUDE** | N 39° 55' 10" |
| **LONGITUDE** | W 105° 40' 40" |

# 10
# GENEVA PARK
# CAMPGROUND

> *The Mount Evans Wilderness is just a hike away from Geneva Park.*

**G**ENEVA PARK CAMPGROUND WAS CONSTRUCTED BY Forest Service volunteers in 1981. Not only did they produce a fine campground, but they also chose their site well. The actual site is in a mildly rolling pine forest in the high country of the northern Pike National Forest. A mere 26 campsites are spread over a fair size of woodland. The location is ideal for exploring the Mount Evans Wilderness, which is less than a mile to the east.

At the head of the actual meadow of Geneva Park an unbroken stand of lodgepole pine grows. Their straight trunks, once used as tent poles for the lodges of western Indian tribes, form a beautiful sight when growing in dense stands as they do here at the campground. Most of the trees here don't have any branches on the lower part of their trunk, then they all seem to sprout branches lush with green needles, contrasting with their reddish-brown patterned bark. Their fallen needles lie on the ground, forming a dusky carpet among the scattered stones. I am sorry to report that some of these lodgepoles had to be cut down because of a dwarf mistletoe parasitic infestation, but the vast majority of trees remain to form an attractive landscape for your camping experience.

Cross Smelter Creek on a bridge, then come to the campground. Here, you will see the more open forest and some stumps of the trees that were cut down to keep the forest healthy. In spite of the cutting, the campsites here have adequate shade. These sites are closest to the pump well.

The actual loop begins after the first seven campsites. The road splits off to the right, just past the vault toilet. Campsites beneath the lodgepoles are either higher or lower than the road, depending on the variation of the terrain. As the loop swings around, there are three campsites that lie under the lodgepole and border their own private meadow opposite the campground road. Beyond the meadow campsites, other campsites outside the loop climb up a hill.

## RATINGS

**Beauty:** ☆ ☆ ☆ ☆
**Privacy:** ☆ ☆ ☆
**Spaciousness:** ☆ ☆ ☆
**Quiet:** ☆ ☆ ☆ ☆
**Security:** ☆ ☆ ☆
**Cleanliness:** ☆ ☆ ☆

This is the least used of the three campgrounds in the Geneva Creek valley. It normally doesn't fill on weekends or even most holidays. You should be able to get a campsite here on all but the busiest traditional holidays.

It's only a 15-minute walk to one of the trailheads to the Mount Evans Wilderness; it's a short drive to the other two entry points to the 74,000-acre preserve that was designated one year before Geneva Park Campground came to be. Within the wilderness are two fourteeners and a rare type of arctic tundra, normally found only within the boundaries of the Arctic Circle. Small pools of water form a plant community unlike the normally dry, brittle Colorado alpine tundra. Mountain goats and bighorn sheep are at home here in this challenging environment.

There are three convenient points of entry to the wilderness for Geneva Park campers. Farther up CR 62 is Guanella Pass at 11,669 feet. It's the easiest way to get high. Just south of Geneva Park you will find the Abyss Trail commencement. This trail climbs strenuously along the glacier-carved valley of Scott Gomer Creek for 7 miles to Abyss Lake. The lake lies perched in a cirque, an encircling wall of rock, with Mount Bierstadt on one side and Mount Evans on the other. Farther south on CR 62 is the Threemile Trail. It heads east into the wilderness toward Tahana Mountain and can be used in combination with the Rosalie and Abyss Trails to form a loop, if you don't mind a bit of road walking.

I enjoy camping in varied forest types. At Geneva Park you can have the lodgepole pine camping experience, then go have the Mount Evans Wilderness hiking experience.

## KEY INFORMATION

**ADDRESS:** Geneva Park Campground South Platte Ranger District 19316 Goddard Ranch Court Morrison, CO 80465

**OPERATED BY:** USDA Forest Service, Pike and San Isabel National Forests, Cimarron and Comanche National Grasslands

**INFORMATION:** (303) 275-5610; www.fs.fed.us

**OPEN:** May–October

**SITES:** 26

**EACH SITE:** Picnic table, fire ring

**ASSIGNMENT:** By reservation

**REGISTRATION:** Call (877) 444-6777, visit reserve america.com, or self-register on site

**FACILITIES:** Hand-pump well, vault toilets

**PARKING:** At campsites only

**FEE:** $14 per night, with additional $9 fee added to each phone or Internet reservation

**ELEVATION:** 9,800 feet

**RESTRICTIONS:** *Pets:* On leash only
*Fires:* In fire rings only
*Alcohol:* At campsites only
*Vehicles:* 20 feet
*Other:* 14-day stay limit

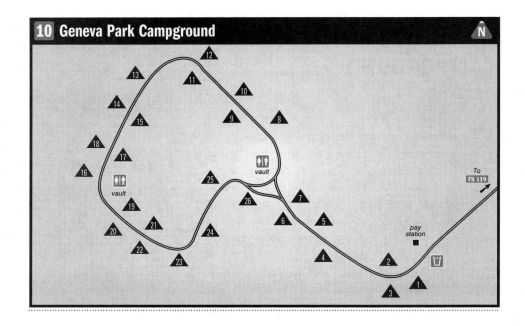

## GETTING THERE

From US 285 in Grant, head north on CR 62 toward Guanella Pass for 6 miles, then veer left on FS 119 and follow it for 0.4 mile to Geneva Park Campground, which will be on your left.

## GPS COORDINATES

**Latitude** N 39° 31' 30.4"
**Longitude** W 105° 44' 17"

# 11
# GOLD PARK CAMPGROUND

**G**OLD PARK IS NEARLY THE IDEAL tent campground. It is somewhat out of the way, on a dirt road, small, well-kept, in a picturesque setting, and adjacent to many outdoor attractions. The dirt road leads up Homestake Valley, a scenic watershed in the Sawatch Range. Gold Park, with only 11 campsites, is located along Homestake Creek, which is hemmed in by Homestake and Whitney Peaks. These mountains are protected as part of the Holy Cross Wilderness. This wilderness area, like most, offers the best recreation of the national forests, mountain biking excepted. Several trailheads are a short drive away. The historic mining town of Holy Cross City is a 4-mile walk, or a rugged four-wheel-drive trip away. Homestake Reservoir and Homestake Creek offer some decent fishing.

*Mine yourself a good time at Gold Park.*

Gold Park is set in a wooded flat between Homestake Creek and a low-lying hill covered in trees and boulders. Beyond the pay station the drive veers to the right, passing the campground host in the first campsite. Lodgepole pines and other smaller conifers shade the entire campground. Large, spacious camping areas are spread along the loop as you proceed up the gravel drive, which then veers left as the rocky hill pinches in the flat toward Homestake Creek.

The campsites come closer to the road as the vehicle turnaround approaches. Three of the best sites are here, one snug against a shaded rock out-crop and the other two lying next to Homestake Creek. These last two sites are the biggest and most coveted sites at Gold Park.

Water spigots and a vault toilet serve this quaint camping area. Gold Park receives moderate use, filling up on the usual holidays. About the only RV you will see here is the campground host. It is unusual, but good, to have a host in a campground this small. The mood here is serene, with the creek providing a naturally symphonic backdrop.

## RATINGS

Beauty: ☆ ☆ ☆ ☆ ☆
Privacy: ☆ ☆ ☆
Spaciousness: ☆ ☆ ☆ ☆ ☆
Quiet: ☆ ☆ ☆ ☆
Security: ☆ ☆ ☆ ☆
Cleanliness: ☆ ☆ ☆ ☆

| | |
|---|---|
| **ADDRESS:** | Gold Park Campground Holy Cross Ranger District 24747 US 24 Minturn, CO 81645 |
| **OPERATED BY:** | USDA Forest Service, White River National Forest |
| **INFORMATION:** | (970) 827-5715; www.fs.fed.us |
| **OPEN:** | May–September |
| **SITES:** | 11 |
| **EACH SITE:** | Picnic table, fire grate |
| **ASSIGNMENT:** | First come, first served; no reservations |
| **REGISTRATION:** | Self-registration on site |
| **FACILITIES:** | Water spigot, vault toilets, trash collection |
| **PARKING:** | At campsites only |
| **FEE:** | $15 per night |
| **ELEVATION:** | 9,300 feet |
| **RESTRICTIONS:** | *Pets:* On leash only *Fires:* In fire grates only *Alcohol:* At campsites only *Vehicles:* 40 feet *Other:* 10-day stay limit |

The upper part of this valley was once home to the mining town of Holy Cross City. The first mines were staked in 1880; Gold Park Mining Company was formed in 1881. The ore assays promised a boom. However, the outer layer of ore proved to be the richest, and the gold wasn't nearly as rich at deeper levels. By 1884, it was finally admitted that the mine was a bust. Another attempt was made in the same area in 1896; a deep tunnel was dug, but the profit just wasn't there. You can take FS 759 up to the site of this mine by foot, bike, or jeep. These days, your only strikes will be from fish on Homestake Creek or Homestake Reservoir, 3 miles up FS 703, your route to Gold Park. The lake is 480 acres in size and brimming with trout.

Take time to explore the Holy Cross Wilderness, whose waters are coveted by Colorado Springs. However, development plans have been halted for the wilderness-that-almost-wasn't due to the city's tampering with the natural flows. Today, you can enjoy the wilderness's alpine lakes and icy streams. The Fall Creek Trail starts about 2 miles up the road to Holy Cross City. The trail heads up to Hunky Dory Lake and the stair-stepping Seven Sisters Lakes, where rock cliffs make for watery backdrops.

It's a 1,500-foot hike in 3 miles on the Missouri Lakes Trail. The trail starts up FS 704 and goes above the timber line. A shorter walk to a high-country lake is the Fancy Pass Trail, which also starts off FS 704 above Gold Park. Pass some dams that you would be seeing all over the place if Colorado Springs had its way, then steeply make your way to Fancy Lake at 2 miles. Treasure Vault Lake is another mile beyond, though you have to go over Fancy Pass, and it is downhill to the lake.

Down from Gold Park is the Whitney Lake Trail, which offers views on its 2.3-mile journey to Whitney Lake. From here you can scale 13,271-foot Mount Whitney, rising on the north shore of the lake, if you follow the west ridge to the top. No matter where you go in the Holy Cross Wilderness, appreciate it, because it almost never came into existence.

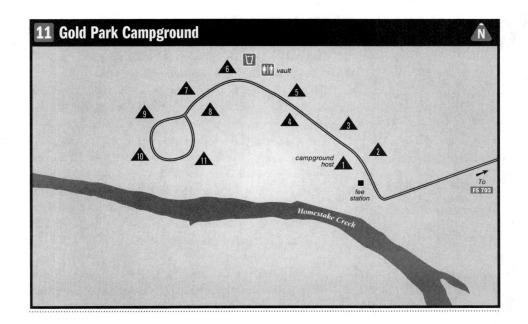

## 11 Gold Park Campground

vault

campground host

fee station

*Homestake Creek*

To FS 703

GETTING THERE

From I-70 near Minturn, head south on US 24 for 11.5 miles to FS 703 (Homestake Road). Turn right on FS 703 and follow it for 7 miles to Gold Park Campground, which will be on your left.

## GPS COORDINATES

| | |
|---|---|
| **LATITUDE** | N 39° 24' 16.0" |
| **LONGITUDE** | W 106° 26' 7.3" |

# 12
# GOLDEN GATE CANYON STATE PARK CAMPGROUND

*This tent-camping getaway is only 30 miles from the Denver metropolitan area.*

**G**OLDEN **G**ATE **IS A PRESERVED SLICE** of the Rocky Mountains just a few minutes away from Denver. Rock spires stand out among rich forests and green meadows. Outstanding views of the Continental Divide can be had to the west. Well-marked and well-maintained trails meander down watery glens to open meadows, where settlements once stood. This refuge is rich in wildlife, from birds to bears. With 55 walk-in tent sites, your camping experience promises to be a good one.

There are two primary campgrounds at Golden Gate Canyon. Reverends Ridge is the big one; it offers spaces for every type of camper. There are ten camp loops of every shape and description, including small circles with parking areas radiating like spokes. There are two loops with pull-through sites for RVs. The old group campground has been converted to six mini-loops that can only be described as different.

But tent campers need only concern themselves with loops F, G, and J in Reverends Ridge; these offer walk-in tent sites. Loops F and G are next to each other. It is a short walk from the parking area to your tent site beneath the lodgepole pines or an aspen grove or two. Loop J is at the very end of the main camping drive, cutting down on drive-by traffic. Some of the campsites are close to the parking area; others are set back in the woods. A stay at Reverends Ridge offers tent campers a compromise: you can stay at the tent sites and still access the water spigots and the hot showers and flush toilets located in the camper services building.

Aspen Meadow is more rustic and the preferred area for tent campers. It has hand-pump wells and vault toilets. But it is also more scenic and isolated from the rest of the campground. Aspen Meadow itself is broken up into three distinctive walk-in tent-camping areas.

The Meadow Loop has 14 campsites in a conifer and aspen wood, next to a large meadow. The sites on

## RATINGS

Beauty: ☆ ☆ ☆
Privacy: ☆ ☆ ☆
Spaciousness: ☆ ☆ ☆
Quiet: ☆ ☆ ☆
Security: ☆ ☆ ☆ ☆ ☆
Cleanliness: ☆ ☆ ☆ ☆

one side of the dirt road are situated amid large boulders that add to the character of the area. The Twin Creek and Conifer Loops are off the ridge in a small valley. The woods are denser here, and a small stream adds to the setting. These are the most popular tent-only sites and are the first to be claimed. Some of the campsites are nearly 100 yards away from the parking area.

The Rimrock Loop has several wooded campsites up on a ridge punctuated with boulder landscaping; these sites offer a view of the lands in the distance and also have the pump well nearest to them. Vault toilets are in each loop at Aspen Meadow.

No matter where you camp, reservations are highly recommended and practically mandatory for summer weekends. Go ahead and make the call to ensure yourself a preferred campsite. Weekdays are not such a problem in this safe, family-oriented campground and natural area.

While you are in the campground, check the notices about ranger programs that are held nightly on weekends. You can learn about the human and natural history of the park in these talks led by park naturalists. There are kids' programs on weekend days that cater specifically to young campers who want to have a good time and learn something about nature without feeling like they are in school.

Other campers will want to strike out on their own on some of the 35 miles of park trails. Everyone should walk the Raccoon Trail. It begins at Panorama Point, where you have a fantastic view of the Continental Divide, and it has interpretive signs to teach hikers a thing or two. The most popular loop hike is the Mountain Lion Trail, which winds for 7 miles into Forgotten Valley, back up a canyon, and up by Windy Peak. Take the side trail to the top of Windy Peak.

The walk into Frazer Meadow is one of the more picturesque park settings. There are three ways to get to the meadow, including the Mule Deer Trail, which connects to Aspen Meadow Campground. There are five ponds in the park and a few small streams that offer trout fishing. Dude's Fishing Hole is very near Aspen Meadow. Denverites and visitors should take advantage of this quick getaway to the real, natural Colorado.

| | |
|---|---|
| **ADDRESS:** | Golden Gate Canyon State Park 92 Crawford Gulch Road Golden, CO 80403 |
| **OPERATED BY:** | Colorado State Parks |
| **INFORMATION:** | (303) 582-3707 or (303) 642-3856 in the summer; parks.state.co.us |
| **OPEN:** | Aspen Meadow, all year; Reverends Ridge, May–Oct. |
| **SITES:** | 55 walk-in tent sites, 86 other |
| **EACH SITE:** | Picnic table, fire grate, tent pad |
| **ASSIGNMENT:** | By reservation or on site |
| **REGISTRATION:** | (800) 678-CAMP (2267) or (303) 470-1144 in Denver, at entrance station or park office, or online at colorado stateparks.reserve america.com, or by a direct link on the park's website |
| **FACILITIES:** | Hot showers, flush and vault toilets, laundry, phone, vending; 28 sites have electricity |
| **PARKING:** | At campsites or walk-in tent campers parking area |
| **FEE:** | $7 Parks Pass plus $16–$18 per night; an additional $10 fee added to each Internet or phone reservation |
| **ELEVATION:** | 9,100 feet |
| **RESTRICTIONS:** | *Pets:* On leash only *Fires:* In fire grates only *Alcohol:* 3.2% beer only *Vehicles:* 40 feet *Other:* 14-day stay limit in 45-day period |

## GETTING THERE

From Golden, take CO 93 north for 1 mile to Golden Gate Canyon Rd. Turn left and follow Golden Gate Canyon Rd. for 15 miles to park.

## GPS COORDINATES

| | |
|---|---|
| **LATITUDE** | N 39° 50' 7.4" |
| **LONGITUDE** | W 105° 25' 6.0" |

# 13
# HERMIT PARK OPEN SPACE:
## KRUGER CAMPGROUND

**K**RUGER CAMPGROUND IS LOCATED IN LARIMER County's Hermit Park Open Space. Hermit Park is a relatively new park (it opened in 2008) approximately 2 miles southeast of Estes Park. I must admit that Kruger Campground is adjacent to one of my favorite new hikes in the area. Kruger Rock Trail is easy to find and a good lung buster. Much of the trail offers a rarely seen perspective of Rocky Mountain National Park, and the views are worth the trip alone.

The campground is just a part of the tidy area that was once a retreat for a private corporation. The cabins are adorable, and the tent campsites are top-notch. RV sites are thrown in for good measure. However, the entire place is laid out for maximum enjoyment of this beautiful piece of mountain real estate. Those corporate folks sure know how to conceptualize and execute a master plan!

Hermit Park Open Space is nestled in hills dotted with wildflowers in the summer and always alive with green amid the plentiful ponderosa pine trees. The starting elevation here is 7,880 feet with an elevation gain on the Kruger Rock hike of more than 1,000 feet, topping out the park at 8,964 feet. Kruger Campground is labeled as campground 3, with a network of notable camping spots as neighbors. Hermit's Hollow Campground (campground 1) has 28 non-electric campsites; Bobcat Campground (campground 2) has 39 non-electric campsites; Granite Gulch Campground (campground 4) is a group camping area; and 15 camper cabins are scattered throughout the park.

To enter the small, private Kruger Campground, pass the Kruger Rock Trail on the right and the Kruger Rock Trail Parking Area and the Bobcat Campground entrance on the left. Enter the loop, where campsites K1–K8 are spaced with ample room and a variety of views. K1 is the first site on the right side and is closest

> *The historic Hermit Park is a new park southeast of Estes Park and close to Rocky Mountain National Park.*

## RATINGS

Beauty: ☆ ☆ ☆ ☆
Privacy: ☆ ☆ ☆ ☆
Spaciousness: ☆ ☆ ☆ ☆
Quiet: ☆ ☆ ☆ ☆
Security: ☆ ☆ ☆ ☆
Cleanliness: ☆ ☆ ☆ ☆

# KEY INFORMATION

**ADDRESS:** Hermit Park Open Space 17 Hermit Park Rd. Estes Park, CO 80517

**OPERATED BY:** Larimer County

**INFORMATION:** (970) 679-4570; larimer.org/parks

**OPEN:** Mar. 1–Dec. 20

**SITES:** 8

**EACH SITE HAS:** Fire grate, picnic table

**ASSIGNMENT:** By reservation

**REGISTRATION:** (800) 397-7795 or larimercamping .com

**FACILITIES:** Comfort station, dump station, picnic shelter, picnic tables, ranger station, drinking water

**PARKING:** At sites or additional parking area

**FEE:** $24 per night, plus $7 entrance permit, plus reservation fee

**ELEVATION:** 7,880 feet

**RESTRICTIONS:** *Pets:* Leashed *Fires:* In designated grates only *Alcohol:* 3.2% beer permitted, glass prohibited *Vehicles:* 30 feet *Other:* 2-night stay required for weekends; 3-night stay required for holidays

to the main road. The next site, on the left, is site K3. Almost directly across from K3 is K2 on the right. Site K2 is located in a private T off the main loop.

Immediately before the loop curves to the left, the restrooms are on the right side. Site K4 is next, also on the right side. Farther down is K5 on the left side and almost directly in the middle of this particular campground loop. Next on the left is an additional restroom. On the right side is K6, which feels as though it is the farthest out and least crowded of all the Kruger sites. Around the next bend and toward the exit of the loop are K7 on the left and K8 on the right.

Many people come to Hermit Park Open Space from the Front Range to relax or hike. Visitors also use the open space as a jumping-off point for Estes Park and the fun of Rocky Mountain National Park. The town of Estes Park is approximately 2 miles northwest of Hermit Park. The Kruger Rock Trail offers unique views of Longs Peak, the Estes Valley, and the Continental Divide. The Homestead Meadows Connector Trail is an easy connector trail for hikers, mountain bikers, and horseback riders to access Homestead Meadows. This 1-mile trail goes to the U.S. Forest Service boundary and 12 miles of trails.

A group pavilion is unique to the Hermit Park Open Space. A 40-acre picnic area with covered pavilion, volleyball court, horseshoe pits, and picnic tables accommodates up to 250 people. Many in the area use the site for special events such as weddings, family reunions, or company picnics.

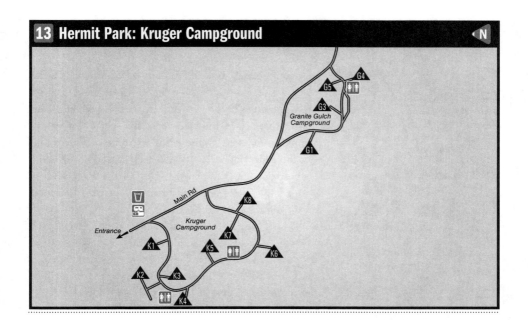

## GETTING THERE

From Denver, take I-25 north to CO 66 and travel west on CO 66 for 16 miles to Lyons. Turn right onto West Main Street onto CO 36 west. Continue on CO 36 for 16.7 miles. The entrance to Hermit Park is on the left.

## GPS COORDINATES

| | |
|---|---|
| **LATITUDE** | N 40° 21' 22" |
| **LONGITUDE** | W 105° 27' 25" |

14
# JACKS GULCH CAMPGROUND

> *Jacks Gulch is the forest campground of the future. It has a little bit of something for everyone, including ten attractive walk-in tent sites.*

**J**ACKS GULCH IS A MODEL CAMPGROUND in many respects. It has separate camping areas for separate types of campers, including RV, horse, and tent campers. No one intrudes on each other's space and a good time is had by all. One thing the Forest Service could not improve on is the natural setting for Jacks Gulch. It is simply beautiful: a huge flat with a mixed forest of ponderosa pine and aspen, interspersed with flower-laden meadows. Many of the tent sites are on the edge of a lovely meadow. The Forest Service did, however, tastefully integrate the campground into this attractive environment.

Enter Jacks Gulch Campground on the main road. Off to your right is the Equestrian Camp. There are five sites with the same amenities as the regular campsites, except they each have a minicorral for the horses. The sites are large and spread farther apart than the average campsites. The two group campgrounds are also over this way.

Veer left, then stay straight and come to the Yarrow Loop. Nice campsites with the newest grills, grates, tent pads, and picnic tables add to the naturally appealing setting. All manner of campers can enjoy this loop, where most of the campsites are shaded by large ponderosa pines.

The other loop is the Columbine Loop; it weaves around like a snake. The campsites have electrical hookups in addition to the standard amenities. This is the home of the big rigs. Splintering off this loop, however, is the walk-in tent camper's area. There is a water spigot and vault toilet in the parking area for tent campers to use. Follow a little gravel path away from the parking area into an aspen wood mixed with some conifers. The campsites themselves splinter off from the main gravel path on a gravel path of their own. Each campsite is far from its neighbor. It's almost like each site is its own

## RATINGS

Beauty: ✩ ✩ ✩ ✩ ✩
Privacy: ✩ ✩ ✩ ✩
Spaciousness: ✩ ✩ ✩ ✩ ✩
Quiet: ✩ ✩ ✩ ✩
Security: ✩ ✩ ✩ ✩
Cleanliness: ✩ ✩ ✩ ✩

miniature campground. I highly recommend this tent-camping experience.

The first five sites have a path of their own, and the second five campsites have their own path as well. Each of these paths connects to the gravel Campground Loop Trail, which makes for a good morning leg-stretcher.

Up Flowers Road beyond the campground is the Flowers Trail. You may have to walk part of the four-wheel-drive road to get to it. After intersecting Beaver Park, enter the Comanche Peaks Wilderness. Elk roam this wilderness, which is also known for its fishing. Leave Beaver Park and climb up to Browns Lake. This path was an old wagon trail in the 1800s.

Little Beaver Creek Trail and Fish Creek Trail enter the wilderness just a little south of the campground on CR 44H. Both make moderate ascents up their respective watersheds and offer trout fishing for hikers and horseback riders. Other trails enter the wilderness from forest roads south of Jacks Gulch. Consult your Arapaho and Roosevelt National Forest map, which you should buy before coming to Jacks Gulch. Not too far south is the northern border of Rocky Mountain National Park, which can be accessed by foot from Pingree Park up the Mummy Pass Trail.

You can also make Jacks Gulch a base camp for recreating in the Poudre Canyon. Rafters, kayakers, and anglers are seen in and around the river, testing the waters. This campground is much more desirable than those in the canyon, yet it is only 6 miles from the canyon and river. You can leave the crowded canyon with its roadside campgrounds and return to Jacks Gulch, where the scene is much quieter and the camping is some of the best in the state.

## KEY INFORMATION

**ADDRESS:** Jacks Gulch Campground Canyon Lakes Ranger District 2150 Centre Ave., Building E Fort Collins, CO 80526

**OPERATED BY:** USDA Forest Service, Arapaho and Roosevelt National Forests, Pawnee National Grassland

**INFORMATION:** (970) 295-6700; www.fs.fed.us

**OPEN:** May 19–Nov. 13

**SITES:** 10 walk-in tent only, 5 equestrian, 55 other

**EACH SITE:** Picnic table, fire grate, stand-up grill, tent pad

**ASSIGNMENT:** First come, first served; no reservations

**REGISTRATION:** Register with host

**FACILITIES:** Water spigots, vault toilets, some sites have electricity

**PARKING:** At campsites and walk-in tent parking area

**FEE:** $18 per night

**ELEVATION:** 8,100 feet

**RESTRICTIONS:** *Pets:* On leash only; see Web for specific horse restrictions
*Fires:* In fire grates
*Alcohol:* At sites
*Vehicles:* 50 feet
*Other:* 14-day limit

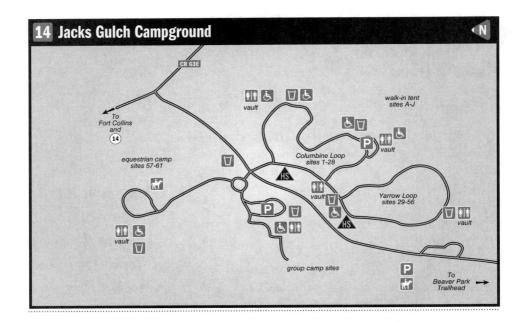

## GETTING THERE

From Fort Collins, drive 10 miles north on US 287 to CO 14. Turn left on CO 14 (Poudre Canyon Highway) and follow it for 24 miles to CR 63E (Pingree Park Road). You will see a sign for Pingree Park. Turn left on CR 63E and follow it for 6 miles to Jacks Gulch Campground, which will be on your right.

## GPS COORDINATES

**LATITUDE** N 40° 37' 35.0"
**LONGITUDE** W 105° 31' 43.0"

# 15
# LONGS PEAK
## CAMPGROUND

**L**ONGS PEAK CAMPGROUND OFFERS THE BEST and worst of the American national park system. This tents-only camping area is located in a scenic setting adjacent to some of the most beautiful mountain land in the Rockies. There are many sights to see and things to do, but the very things that attract you to this park also attract many other visitors.

Longs Peak is an extremely popular hike here. Cars will line the road leading to the trailhead and campground. It takes a combination of timing and luck to get a campsite during the peak season, which is from late June through mid-September. When you do get a campsite, you will realize that in spite of all the cars nearby, the hustle and bustle won't overwhelm you in this 26-site campground. The trailhead parking area, however, will have all the hustle and bustle.

Pass the line of parked cars along Longs Peak Road and come to a split in the road. Turn right and enter the campground. To your left is the always-full-in-summer trailhead parking. The teardrop-shaped, gravel campground loop makes its way beneath a lodgepole woodland pocked with boulders and smaller trees. The sites are mostly on the outside of the loop and have somewhat obstructed views of the Twin Sisters peaks across the Tahosa Valley in the Roosevelt National Forest.

More campsites are stretched along the peak side of the loop. As popular as they are, they are well maintained. A hill rises against the campground. This is the campground's rockier side; campsites are more spread out over here. Overall, the sites are average in size, with ample room for the average tent. But always being full does make the place seem a bit confined. Colorful tents and colorful people give Longs Peak some extra pizzazz.

Water spigots are situated around the campground, but there is only one toilet for each gender located in the center of the campground. You might have to wait in line

> *This tent-only campground can be your base camp for exploring the east side of Rocky Mountain National Park.*

## RATINGS

**Beauty:** ✰ ✰ ✰
**Privacy:** ✰ ✰
**Spaciousness:** ✰ ✰ ✰
**Quiet:** ✰ ✰
**Security:** ✰ ✰ ✰ ✰
**Cleanliness:** ✰ ✰ ✰ ✰

## KEY INFORMATION

**ADDRESS:** Longs Peak
Campground
Rocky Mountain
National Park
Estes Park, CO
80517

**OPERATED BY:** National Park Service; Rocky Mountain National Park

**information:** (970) 586-1206;
nps.gov/romo

**open:** All year

**SITES:** 26

**EACH SITE:** Picnic table, fire grate, tent pad

**ASSIGNMENT:** First come, first served; no reservations

**REGISTRATION:** Self-registration on site

**FACILITIES:** Water spigot, flush toilets (no water October–May)

**PARKING:** At campsites only

**FEE:** $20 per night (Memorial Day–mid-September) or $14 in the off season when the water is shut off; plus a separate park entrance fee applies

**ELEVATION:** 9,400 feet

**restriction:** *Pets:* On leash only
*Fires:* In fire grates only
*Alcohol:* At campsites only
*Vehicles:* No RVs
*Other:* 7 nights per campsite June–September; 14-night limit in winter

for that too. Realistically, you will feel lucky and appreciative when you do get a campsite; despite the crowds, you'll still have a pleasurable tent camping experience here. Try to visit during the shoulder seasons—June or late September—when you can get a campsite much easier. Bring your own water and a warm sleeping bag if you come in winter.

I recommend auto-touring the park your first day, maybe doing some shorter hikes, then tackling Longs Peak first thing the next morning, when you have all day to make the climb. Driving Trail Ridge Road is a must. It is a rite of passage at Rocky Mountain National Park. The views are as exhilarating as the air is cold up there. Then check out the exhibits and self-guided nature trail at Moraine Park Museum. Back at Longs Peak, take a warm-up hike on the Storm Pass Trail. It leads up to the Eugenia Mine Site and onto Storm Pass after 2.5 miles.

Then go to bed early. Your route to the top of Longs Peak will be the Keyhole Route, which is generally free of snow from mid-July until mid-September. The final part of the route is 1.6 miles beyond the end of the maintained trail; most of the scramble is marked on the rock below you.

The park service recommends that you try to leave the trailhead between 3 a.m. and 6 a.m. to make the 7.5 miles to the summit of Longs Peak by noon. Bad weather can arise at any time, but it is more likely in the afternoon during the summer. Bring plenty of warm clothes and lung power. The round-trip lasts 12–15 hours. Be sure to keep your campsite a second night because you will be too exhausted to do anything except make supper and hit the sack.

Just a few miles south of Longs Peak is the Wild Basin area, a quieter section of the park's east side. Many old-time Rocky Mountain enthusiasts consider this to be the best area of the park. Many watery features in the basin make great day hikes. It is only 0.3 mile from the ranger station in Wild Basin to Copeland Falls. Calypso Cascades is 1.8 miles up where Saint Vrain Creek splits. Ouzel Falls is 2.7 miles up the trail from the ranger station. Continue a little farther to see the peaks above and the plains below. There are several alpine lakes to access in Wild Basin.

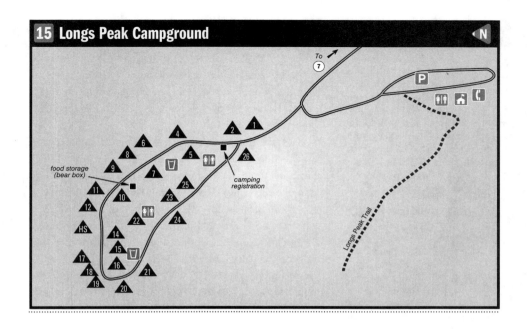

food storage
(bear box)

camping
registration

Longs Peak Trail

## GETTING THERE

From Estes Park, head south
on CO 7 for 8 miles to Longs
Peak Road. Turn right on
Longs Peak Road and follow
it for 3 miles to Longs Peak
Campground, which will be
on your right.

## GPS COORDINATES

| | |
|---|---|
| **LATITUDE** | N 40° 16' 29.5" |
| **LONGITUDE** | W 105° 33' 9.0" |

> *Lost Park is your camping ticket to the Lost Creek Wilderness.*

**L**OST PARK CAMPGROUND SITS ATOP A knoll in the large valley at the confluence of Indian Creek, North Fork Lost Creek, and South Fork Lost Creek. The Kenosha and Tarryall Mountains serve as your campground cathedrals. It is in this enhanced setting that you can set up your tent, then fish, hike, and explore the Lost Creek Wilderness until the call of civilization is too loud to ignore.

You won't want to leave this small, hilltop campground cloaked in lodgepole pines and complemented by other conifers. With only 12 campsites and nearly 20 miles of dirt road, civilization doesn't exactly come knocking on your tent flap. Two drives with vehicle turnarounds at their ends divide the campsites, which are spread very far apart.

The first drive circles the top of the knoll. Most of the campsites are on the more heavily wooded left side, while the few on the right look over Lost Creek below and Bison Peak above. A campsite lies in the rocky center of the auto turnaround. Other boulders serve as landscaping car barriers.

The lower drive turns left and drops toward the North Fork of Lost Creek. Two campsites lie on a slope to your left. Stay here if you don't mind sleeping a little tilted. Pass the northbound section of the Brookside-McCurdy Trail. Follow the drive as it swings right along the creek, passing the well pump in a meadow and a lonesome campsite on your right that offers the maximum in privacy. The drive continues past other campsites that sit on a small hill looking downstream on Lost Creek. These sites also have other conifers in addition to the lodgepole. Then you come to the vehicle turnaround with one more large campsite on your right.

There is one set of vault toilets for each gender at each loop. But bigger amenities, such as three fishable streams and three trailheads at the campground, will

## RATINGS

Beauty: ✿ ✿ ✿ ✿
Privacy: ✿ ✿ ✿ ✿
Spaciousness: ✿ ✿ ✿ ✿
Quiet: ✿ ✿ ✿ ✿
Security: ✿ ✿ ✿
Cleanliness: ✿ ✿ ✿

make you appreciate Lost Park more than anything else. The Lost Creek Wilderness, which is most of the land you see around you, is almost 120,000 acres of meadows, woods, and unusual granite formations, where one of Colorado's largest herds of bighorn sheep live. There are nearly 100 miles of trails to enjoy, and you can probably get most of the hiking you desire without restarting your vehicle until it is time to head home. After all, a wilderness is defined as an untrammeled place where man is just a visitor. And visit you must.

The Wigwam Trail heads east along Lost Creek proper. Soon you'll come to the very large East Lost Park. This is a huge meadow that goes on and on. Veer right on an unmaintained fishing trail if you want to keep going down Lost Creek. The Wigwam Trail follows a feeder stream up and over a divide to the Wigwam Creek drainage.

The north end of the Brookside-McCurdy Trail skirts the wilderness; mountain bikers can pedal this section. It then intersects the Colorado Trail, where you can veer right into the wilderness high country or veer left and keep on biking to the top, over to the Craig Creek drainage. If you go south on the Brookside-McCurdy Trail from the campground, you will head up Indian Creek toward Bison Pass. There are fishable waters with small but spunky trout ready to tear at your lure on all the creeks.

Mountain bikers can't enter the wilderness, but they have their own trails to use just back down FS 56. Walleye Gulch Road and Topaz Road, FS 854 and FS 446, respectively, can be used with other connecting Forest Service roads to make loops. I recommend that hikers, bikers, and anglers all get the Trails Illustrated map titled *Tarryall Mountains, Kenosha Pass,* for the general area (maps.nationalgeographic.com/trails). Get all your supplies before you get anywhere near the area; Lost Park is far from the main roads. The nearby towns are small and don't have much in the way of supplies except for the convenience store variety. One more thing, bring your binoculars to help you spot bighorn sheep.

## KEY INFORMATION

| | |
|---|---|
| **ADDRESS:** | Lost Park Campground South Park Ranger District P.O. Box 219 320 Highway 285 Fairplay, CO 80440 |
| **OPERATED BY:** | USDA Forest Service, Pike and San Isabel National Forests, Cimarron and Comanche National Grasslands |
| **INFORMATION:** | (719) 836-2031; www.fs.fed.us |
| **OPEN:** | May–September |
| **SITES:** | 12 |
| **EACH SITE:** | Picnic table, fire grate |
| **ASSIGNMENT:** | First come, first served; no reservations |
| **REGISTRATION:** | Self-registration on site |
| **FACILITIES:** | Hand-pump well, vault toilets |
| **PARKING:** | At campsites only |
| **FEE:** | $10 per night |
| **ELEVATION:** | 10,000 feet |
| **RESTRICTIONS:** | *Pets:* On leash only *Fires:* In fire grates only *Alcohol:* At campsites only *Vehicles:* 22 feet *Other:* 14-day stay limit |

## 16 Lost Park Campground

## GETTING THERE

From Jefferson, drive north 1 mile to CR 56 (Lost Park Road), turn right, and drive east for 19 miles to the dead end at Lost Park Campground.

## GPS COORDINATES

**LATITUDE** N 39° 17' 4.0"
**LONGITUDE** W 105° 30 22.0"

# 17
# LOWER NARROWS CAMPGROUND

**T**HE POUDRE (PRONOUNCED: POOH-DER) RIVER IS full of plenty of river lore and conjures up images of French trappers hooting down fierce rapids in the canyon. Its official name is Cache la Poudre River, and legend has it that the river was named when a party of westward fur trappers was forced to lighten its load near the banks after being caught in a heavy snowfall. The order was given to *cache la poudre* or "hide the powder" so that it could be retrieved the following spring. The Poudre River, with it's designation as a Wild and Scenic River, is quite wild. In heavy runoff years, we've rafted sections of the river that spilled us in and claimed this author, hooting and hollering, bobbing along, until pulled back inside our boat. Luckily I emerged unscathed, but the river earns quick respect from those who recreate here. One area that is sacred is a section called the Narrows: a narrow cleft where the river has cut through the rock walls. Even driving through this area is dicey, with hairpin turns, blind spots, and looming canyon walls. If I want a good scare, we park and look at the river during the spring, when the water is crashing down, full of the cold, spring runoff. The Class VI rapids tear into the canyon walls and pummel anything in their path. A few crazies and experienced kayakers have been known to run these rapids and live to tell. (River rapids are usually rated on a raftable scale starting at I, considered easy, and ending at V, considered not so easy. So you get the idea of what a VI means.)

The Narrows Campgrounds, both Upper and Lower, are located just above said rapids. From the Lower Narrows Campground, you can walk a half mile to witness the gnarly area previously described.

Poudre Canyon recreationists are usually limited to RV-clogged camping areas, with one exception. The Lower Narrows is the tent-only portion of the Narrows Campground, complete with a separate entrance, and

> *The Lower Narrows, right on a wild river, is the best tent camping in the canyon.*

## RATINGS

Beauty: ✩ ✩ ✩
Privacy: ✩ ✩ ✩
Spaciousness: ✩ ✩ ✩
Quiet: ✩ ✩ ✩
Security: ✩ ✩ ✩ ✩
Cleanliness: ✩ ✩ ✩ ✩ ✩

**ADDRESS:** Lower Narrows
Canyon Lakes
Ranger District
2150 Centre Ave.,
Building E
Fort Collins, CO
80526

**OPERATED BY:** USDA Forest Ser-
vice, Arapaho and
Roosevelt National
Forests, Pawnee
National Grassland

**INFORMATION:** (970) 295-6700;
www.fs.fed.us

**OPEN:** May–October

**SITES:** 8

**EACH SITE:** Fire grate, picnic
table, tent pad

**ASSIGNMENT:** By reservation

**REGISTRATION:** By phone (877)
444-6777, online at
www.reserveusa
.com, or self-regis-
tration on site

**FACILITIES:** Vault toilets, drinking water (usually
turned off at the
end of September)

**PARKING:** Lot for exactly
8 cars

**FEE:** $17 (half price
when water is not
available), an addi-
tional $9 fee added
to each Internet or
phone reservation

**ELEVATION:** 6,400 feet

**RESTRICTIONS:** *Pets:* On leash
*Fires:* In grates
*Alcohol:* Allowed
*Vehicles:* Passenger
vehicles only
*Other:* 8 people per
site

is by far the best tent camping in the canyon. There is plenty of hiking, especially in the nearby Comanche Peak Wilderness. Anglers, off-road enthusiasts, and Sunday drivers all clog the roadway, especially during the summer weekends, but all seem to be having a great time. The Poudre River is the main draw to the Narrows Campgrounds, and the Lower Narrows campsites are as close as you can get to sleeping on shore, especially preferred sites 12 and 13. Site 14 is a good second choice, and site 11 isn't bad either but is a little higher from the river. Light sleepers take note: the river rages through here in May and June with accompanying noise.

Lower Narrows Campground is configured as a loop. At the entrance, take a right turn to start a counterclockwise loop. Numbering starts at site 8 since Lower Narrows and Upper Narrows are managed jointly by the ranger district at the Narrows Campground. Park at the parking lot right next to site 8. There is an obvious disadvantage to being near the parking lot. Site 8, along with sites 9 and 10 are closer to the road. Sites 11–15 are scattered about from here. As mentioned before, sites 12 and 13 are most popular, with 14 not far behind, and sites 11 and 15 earning honorable mentions.

Even in other months this is not a sleepy stretch of river, but a rather steep and rocky section, as is most of Poudre Canyon. The river may be boated by experienced rafters and kayakers above this area and again resuming at Stevens Gulch, 2.5 miles downstream. Between the campground and Stevens Gulch are the several Class VI drops hidden from the road. Lower Narrows Campground is a good alternative to the high-use, RV-type campgrounds in the area. There are very few services for miles in either direction except for a few seasonal stores. If you are interested in rafting or kayaking, the Poudre River is open to both private and commercial boaters. We have our own gear, but would recommend setting up an outfitted trip in Fort Collins before heading out.

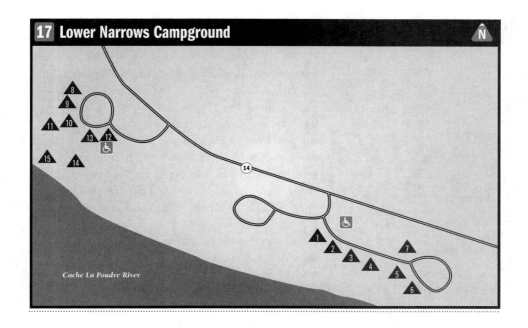

*Cache La Poudre River*

## GETTING THERE

Drive 7 miles north of Fort Collins on US 287. Turn left on CO 14, also known as Poudre Canyon Highway, and drive approximately 16 miles west. If coming from upper Poudre Canyon/ Cameron Pass, look for the entrance just after Narrows Campground.

## GPS COORDINATES

| | |
|---|---|
| **LATITUDE** | N 40° 41' 21.2" |
| **LONGITUDE** | W 105° 25' 57" |

> *The access to Indian Peaks Wilderness and Rocky Mountain National Park is second to none.*

**P**EACEFUL VALLEY AND CAMP DICK HAVE camp hosts buzzing around in golf carts, keeping this tidy campground, tidy. RVs are also in attendance, and summer camp crowds are frequent. So why include this area in a tent-camping book, you ask? Peaceful Valley and Camp Dick are situated in a glacial valley adjacent to Middle St. Vrain Creek. Access to the Indian Peaks Wilderness and Rocky Mountain National Park are second to none and would easily cause a mega-resort to drool over the real estate if there were ever a price put on this priceless acreage. (Don't worry, they can never sell.)

The arrangement of the 58 campsites here is carefully thought out with particular attention paid to placement of the sites tucked into the wooded landscape. All campers live in harmony here, especially those confined to the smaller sites. RV campers may also convert to smaller accommodations after they see what amazing spots are allowed for tent campers here.

Technically two campgrounds, Peaceful Valley and Camp Dick are connected by a short road and appear to be one and the same. The access to scenery and recreational opportunities in Indian Peaks Wilderness and Rocky Mountain National Park is the reason to be here. Hiking can even be directly accessed from the St. Vrain Trailhead at the west end of the campground. Backpackers, horseback riders, mountain bikers, four-wheel-drive users, and anglers all enjoy the advantages of the surroundings. Since Indian Peaks is a wilderness area, those wanting to camp there or recreate in the wilderness boundary should contact the Boulder Ranger District regarding specific regulations that apply. The same goes for Rocky Mountain National Park, so contact the National Park Service for rules particular to that area. It's important to note that without entering the wilderness or national park, there is plenty to do. The campground itself is still in the national forests.

## RATINGS

**Beauty:** ☆ ☆ ☆ ☆
**Privacy:** ☆ ☆ ☆
**Spaciousness:** ☆ ☆ ☆ ☆
**Quiet:** ☆ ☆ ☆
**Security:** ☆ ☆ ☆ ☆
**Cleanliness:** ☆ ☆ ☆ ☆

Peaceful Valley and Camp Dick have been remodeled recently, and the biggest improvement is the paved road that cuts down on dust creeping into the campsites. Some sites at Peaceful Valley and Camp Dick are not recommended during peak season because of privacy and the fact that they are essentially set up for RVs. But the cream of the crop, mentioned here, are nice, especially if you can get here during the week. Of the 58 campsites, we have made a list of the top ten. By far the best for privacy and space is Camp Dick site 35 at the end of a loop. Camp Dick sites 10, 12, 15, 16, 18, 19, 40, and 41 are also recommended for space and privacy. Peaceful Valley site 1 is the final pick because a slight embankment provides extra privacy, and it is also right on the edge of the Middle St. Vrain Creek. Although we've narrowed the choices, keep in mind that all campsites are scattered among the spruce, pine, and aspen trees, and all have tent pads, parking, and fire areas.

Enter Peaceful Valley first, cross Middle St. Vrain Creek, and site 7 is directly to the left. A right turn takes you into a nice, small loop that starts with our favorite site, 1; circles counterclockwise to 2, 3, 4, 5, and 6; and then deposits you back to site 7. Continue to site 8, which is usually the host site; site 9 is on the right, next to the drinking water. A cluster of sites—10, 11, 12, 13, and 14—are on the left. Across from them is site 9, and next to that is site 15. Site 16 is also on this right side, and site 17 is the last on the left. Sites 8–17 should actually receive high honorable mention because they have dense trees and more shelter than sites 1–7.

Leave Peaceful Valley and enter into Camp Dick. On the right are sites 1 through 9, which are quite close together and have few trees or little privacy. However, favorite sites 40 and 41 are on the left and are very different with tons of privacy and beautiful scenery. Continue toward the right and pass sites 10 and 12, which are favorites; 11, 13, and 14 come next; and a small loop begins with favorites 15, 16, curves to an okay 17, and then comes back to two more favorites, 18 and 19. Sites 20, 21, 22, and 23 are on the right side of a new loop; sites 24, 26, and 28 are inside the loop and not recommended. Sites 26 and 27 are on the opposite side. Site 26 wasn't a favorite because it sits in the open, and site 27 is very close

**ADDRESS:** Peaceful Valley and Camp Dick Boulder Ranger District 2140 Yarmouth Avenue Boulder, CO 80301

**OPERATED BY:** USDA Forest Service, Arapaho and Roosevelt National Forests, Pawnee National Grassland

**INFORMATION:** (303) 541-2500; www.fs.fed.us

**OPEN:** Mid-May–mid-Oct.

**SITES:** 58 (Camp Dick, 41; Peaceful Valley, 17)

**EACH SITE:** Picnic table, fire ring, upright grill, tent pad

**ASSIGNMENT:** By reservation

**REGISTRATION:** By phone (877) 444-6777, online at reserveusa.com, or self-registration on site

**FACILITIES:** Water, vault toilets

**PARKING:** At campsite

**FEE:** $17 per night, $20 for oversized sites, an additional $9 fee added to each Internet or phone reservation

**ELEVATION:** 8,650 feet

**RESTRICTIONS:** *Pets:* On leash
*Fires:* In designated areas
*Alcohol:* Allowed
*Vehicles:* 55 feet
*Other:* 14-day stay limit; maximum 8–12 people per site, varies by site

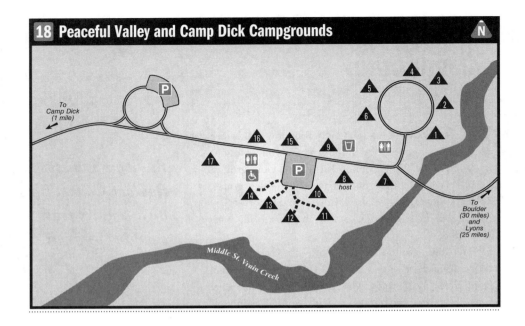

## GETTING THERE

Peaceful Valley Campground is off CO 72 (also known as the Peak to Peak Highway) at mile marker 50, approximately 19 miles north of Nederland and 20 miles south of Estes Park. It may also be accessed via CO 66 west to Lyons, then southwest on CO 7 for approximately 12 miles to CO 72, and south on CO 72 approximately 4 miles.

to the vault toilet. As the loop ends, a straightaway hosts ten honorable mention sites. On the right are sites 29–34, and on the left are sites 39–36. Site 35 is at the far end of all of these sites—so far at the end of the turnaround loop, in fact, that it's our #1 pick.

This area was once the site of a Civilian Conservation Corps camp, established in the 1930s. Now, the campground is open to all and is normally full for the weekend by early Friday afternoon. So, plan to arrive early, consider making a reservation, and always try to take time off during the week to really take advantage of this beautiful place.

## GPS COORDINATES

LATITUDE N 40° 7' 57"
LONGITUDE W 105° 30' 32"

**T**HE LAST COUPLE OF MILES TO Rainbow Lakes are bone-jarringly bumpy. But once here you'll wonder why you haven't come sooner. It is an old campground that has received a makeover. The picnic tables, grates, and grills have been replaced; however, the Forest Service did cap the water well, so now you must bring your own water.

The campground is just south of Rocky Mountain National Park and is adjacent to the equally scenic Indian Peaks Wilderness. The forest here is upper-level montane, primarily lodgepole, with some Engelmann spruce and a few aspens struggling to survive. On my late June visit, the aspens had barely started leafing out. Their short growth time coincides with the short time this campground is open.

If you are in the area, stay here. The Rainbow Lakes are only half a mile from the campground. Make your visit up to the lakes for the day, and camp down at the campground. That preserves the natural resource and concentrates your impact at the campground. Rainbow Lakes Campground can also be a base camp for exploring the east side of Rocky Mountain National Park. Be forewarned: this campground receives heavy weekend use in late summer.

Rainbow Lakes Campground lies along a stream emanating from the Rainbow Lakes that feed into Caribou Creek. Willows and beaver ponds break up the meadow to your left; on your right is a rising woodland. The first three sites are on a spur to your right. One is a pull-through site, but don't expect to find RVers up here unless they enjoy tearing up their rig. Continue up the main drive and another loop spurs off your right. It contains six campsites that are beneath conifers. The two sites inside the spur loop are a little small.

The rest of the campsites border the stream and are spread apart well beneath the trees. The last campsite is

> *Rainbow Lakes is Boulder County's best high-country tent camping getaway.*

## RATINGS

Beauty: ✪ ✪ ✪ ✪
Privacy: ✪ ✪ ✪
Spaciousness: ✪ ✪ ✪ ✪
Quiet: ✪ ✪ ✪ ✪
Security: ✪ ✪ ✪
Cleanliness: ✪ ✪ ✪

# KEY INFORMATION

**ADDRESS:** Rainbow Lakes Campground Boulder Ranger District 2140 Yarmouth Avenue Boulder, CO 80301

**OPERATED BY:** USDA Forest Service, Arapaho and Roosevelt National Forests, Pawnee National Grassland

**INFORMATION:** (303) 541-2500; www.fs.fed.us

**OPEN:** July–September, sometimes longer

**SITES:** 16

**EACH SITE:** Picnic table, tent pad, fire grate, stand-up grill

**ASSIGNMENT:** First come, first served; no reservations

**REGISTRATION:** Self-registration on-site

**FACILITIES:** Vault toilets (bring water)

**PARKING:** At campsites only

**FEE:** $11 per night

**ELEVATION:** 10,000 feet

**RESTRICTIONS:** *Pets:* On leash only *Fires:* In fire grates only *Alcohol:* At campsites only *Vehicles:* 20 feet *Other:* 14-day stay limit; maximum 8 people allowed per site

away from the others, next to the trailhead parking area for Rainbow Lakes. Three vault toilets for this small campground are overkill, but at least you won't have to walk far to the bathroom no matter where you are camped.

Stated simply, come here during the week or Sunday night if at all possible. Not only is the campground full on weekends, but there is also significant traffic coming through the campground to and from the Rainbow Lakes Trailhead.

From Nederland you drove part of the Peak to Peak Scenic Byway. Continue to enjoy this drive north to Estes Park, where there are supplies, and south to Black Hawk and Central City, where there is legalized gambling. The casinos offer limited-stakes gaming.

However, a sure bet is the Indian Peaks Wilderness next door. The glaciers in the Indian Peaks are the southernmost ones in North America. This high wilderness starts at 10,700 feet. Much of the scenery is austere tundra, rock, and ice. The Rainbow Lakes Trail goes the half mile to the lakes and is a must-hike.

The Arapaho Glacier Trail runs in and out of the wilderness a few miles up to the Arapaho Glacier overlook. The glacier is on this side of North Arapaho Peak. It is 6 miles from the trailhead to the Arapaho Pass Trail. Other trailheads into the busy Indian Peaks lie north off forest roads that intersect the Peak to Peak Byway.

Another area to consider is the Wild Basin of Rocky Mountain National Park. This is a watery place, where many cascades tumble down from the heights and picturesque lakes lie beneath craggy peaks. The basin is north on the Peak to Peak Byway. Get hiking information from the ranger station there.

For a bit of interesting civilization, try the college town of Boulder, 45 minutes down Boulder Canyon. This eclectic place is known for its diversity and beauty. Take a walk down Pearl Street, where the streets are blocked off and the dining, shopping, and culture reigns supreme. Nearby Nederland, albeit a more toned down version of Boulder, earns honorable mention with their few but quality restaurants and a great grocery store. Make a visit to Nederland part of your Rainbow Lakes experience.

P

P
vault

10    9    8    7    6    5    4

11    12    vault    16    15    14

P

vault

beaver
ponds

To
72

## GETTING THERE

From Nederland, drive north
on CO 72 for 6.5 miles to FS
298 (also known as CR 116).
There will be a sign for
University of Colorado
Mountain Research Station.
Turn left on FS 298 and
follow it for 6 miles to Rainbow Lakes Campground.

## GPS COORDINATES

| | |
|---|---|
| **LATITUDE** | N 40° 0' 37.5" |
| **LONGITUDE** | W 105° 34' 16" |

> *A campground escape that is worthy of the outlaw in all of us.*

**R**OBBERS ROOST CONJURES UP IMAGES OF wild-West outlaws and hideouts for bandits that may have just had a shootout at the OK Corral. True to its name, this campground offers plenty of sites to escape to in its dark, wooded terrain and remote location. At the base of Berthoud Pass, far from the buzzing of the I-70 corridor, modern outlaws can find peace and hide out from a nagging boss or mounting bills. Never far from modern comforts, campers at Robbers Roost may also step out and hit the small mountain town of Winter Park.

Robbers Roost is a spread-out campground in the tall timber at the western base of Berthoud Pass. RVs are not officially banned here, but the parking spots are smaller than most and many sites simply can not host a large rig. Robbers Roost is a tried-and-true Colorado mountain campground with a traditional "gather around the campfire in the pines" atmosphere. The dispersed arrangement is perfect for naturalists who don't like a strict layout or cookie-cutter feel at each campsite. The terrain allows for little room at each site and is suitable for small and midsized tents only. Level areas for tents are not in abundance, and it takes some time at each site to scope for the best place to lay your tarp—a refreshing change from the perfectly lined up tent pads at some campgrounds.

Entering the campground and starting a counter-clockwise loop, the road is visible from site 1, but sites 2–6, at the beginning of the campground, immediately eliminate the view of the highway. These five sites are the best in the campground because they are private and spacious. Sites 2 and 3 are best for space and flatness, while site 6 is the favorite because it is more private and at the end of a loop. A small stream passes these five sites, and site 6 even has a small footbridge you cross for campsite access. Site 8 offers less privacy since it's in the middle of the loop. Sites 7, 9, 10, and 11 are on the

## RATINGS

Beauty: ✪ ✪ ✪ ✪
Privacy: ✪ ✪ ✪ ✪
Spaciousness: ✪ ✪ ✪ ✪
Quiet: ✪ ✪ ✪
Security: ✪ ✪ ✪
Cleanliness: ✪ ✪ ✪ ✪

opposite side and uphill of the loop and are okay, but tent space is smallest at these.

Robbers Roost does get a little road noise from US 40, but this is a mountain pass, not a major interstate. This area also receives a huge amount of snow accumulation and typically opens later than the scheduled Memorial Day.

Winter Park and Mary Jane ski areas are just down the road and offer fun all year, such as mountain biking and hiking in the summer camping season. The nearby Moffat Road is an abandoned high-alpine railroad grade, now a dirt road open to cars and bikes. Moffat Road is a fun, lung-buster of a mountain bike ride up to Rollins Pass, and a great cruiser of a ride down. The town of Winter Park is only 10 minutes away from the campground and is a great place to eat, shop, and even catch a movie.

The Sulphur Ranger District, composed of more than 400,000 acres in Grand County, Colorado, is surrounded by mountains, meadows, and lakes. To the west of Robbers Roost, the three lakes of Grand, Granby, and Shadow Mountain are fun for the day with a small boat or fishing pole. The Stillwater area next to Grand Lake has miles of trails for four-wheel-drive enthusiasts.

To the east of Robbers Roost, the ski area on top of Berthoud Pass is permanently closed, but the region offers tons of hiking and access to plenty of wildlife and wildflowers.

The 12,000-13,000-foot mountains above the campground make up the spine of the Continental Divide. The tiny Fraser River that starts in the valley, near Robbers Roost, grows to become the massive Colorado River and flows into the Pacific Ocean to the west.

In contrast, and in the magical allure of the Continental Divide, all precipitation on the other side of the ridge above the campground ends up in tributaries that feed into the Atlantic Ocean to the east. Avalanche shoots on this side of Berthoud Pass are always awe-inspiring, fun to locate, and less threatening during the summer camping season.

## KEY INFORMATION

**ADDRESS:** Robbers Roost Sulphur Ranger District 9 Ten Mile Drive, P.O. Box 10 Granby, CO 80446

**OPERATED BY:** Fraser River Valley Lions Club under an agreement with USDA Forest Service, Arapaho, and Roosevelt National Forests, Pawnee National Grassland

**INFORMATION:** (970) 887-4100; www.fs.fed.us

**OPEN:** Memorial Day–Labor Day; may open later in heavy snow years

**SITES:** 11

**EACH SITE:** Fire grate or fire pit, picnic table

**ASSIGNMENT:** First come, first served

**REGISTRATION:** On site

**FACILITIES:** Vault toilets, no water

**PARKING:** 1 space at each campsite

**FEE:** $12 per night

**ELEVATION:** 9,826 feet

**RESTRICTIONS:** *Pets:* On leash *Fires:* In designated areas *Alcohol:* Allowed *Vehicles:* 25 feet *Other:* 14-day stay limit, 5 people per site with a maximum of 2 tents per site

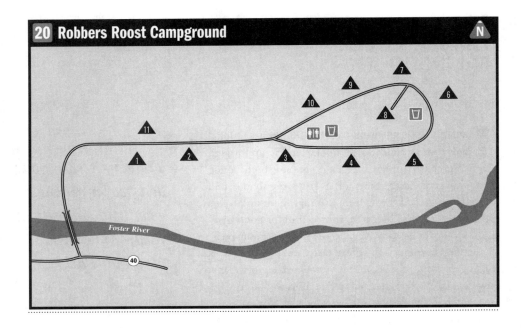

## GETTING THERE

Travel 5 miles south of Winter Park ski area on US 40 to the base of Berthoud Pass.

## GPS COORDINATES

**LATITUDE** N 39° 48' 21"
**LONGITUDE** W 105° 44' 23"

**T**IMBER CREEK REMINDS ME OF AN old-time national park campground: wood smoke curling up through the evergreens; families mingling; couples—both young and old—interacting; tents of every size, shape, and description spread through the campground; and a few pop-up trailers and bigger rigs thrown in for good measure. Everyone is moving at a relaxed, vacation pace. Someone is grilling something tasty, another person is rigging their fishing rod, and yet another is snoozing in a lawn chair. You get the feeling that all is well here.

Timber Creek lies in a wooded flat alongside the headwaters of the Colorado River. Trail Ridge Road forms the other boundary. Lodgepole pine is the primary tree here. Pine needles and an occasional rock form the understory. The campsites are spread out in this sizable campground on a main drive with four loops spurring off it. The odd thing is that the loops are named after trees that don't even grow in this park (dogwood is one example)! The main drive passes the ranger station and passes some large campsites. Just across from the ranger station are the first tent-only campsites. The tent campsites have a car pull-in area, then your campsite is in the woods across planted wood poles separating the camping and parking areas.

The main drive swings alongside the willows of the Colorado River. A few riverside sites are in mixed shade and sun and are the best campsites here. The river and mountain views are nice. The rest of the campground is well shaded by lodgepole pine. The first camping loop splits off to the left and has tent-only and general-use sites. The next loop has tent-only and general-use campsites, also. The third loop has only general campsites, but tenters are the majority here too. The fourth and final loop has mostly tent-only sites.

There are several beaver ponds off in the meadow toward the river. Other wildlife, notably moose and elk,

*Timber Creek is your best bet for getting a good tent campsite in Rocky Mountain National Park.*

## RATINGS

Beauty: ✰ ✰ ✰ ✰
Privacy: ✰ ✰ ✰
Spaciousness: ✰ ✰ ✰
Quiet: ✰ ✰ ✰
Security: ✰ ✰ ✰ ✰ ✰
Cleanliness: ✰ ✰ ✰ ✰ ✰

## KEY INFORMATION

| | |
|---|---|
| **ADDRESS:** | Timber Creek Campground Rocky Mountain National Park Estes Park, CO 80517 |
| **OPERATED BY:** | National Park Service; Rocky Mountain National Park |
| **INFORMATION:** | (970) 586-1206; nps.gov/romo |
| **OPEN:** | All year |
| **SITES:** | 33 tent-only sites, 67 other |
| **EACH SITE:** | Picnic table, fire grate, tent pad |
| **ASSIGNMENT:** | First come, first served; no reservations |
| **REGISTRATION:** | Self-registration on site |
| **FACILITIES:** | Water spigot, flush toilets, phone (no water late Sept.–May) |
| **PARKING:** | At campsites only |
| **FEE:** | $20 per night, $14 in off season (when water is turned off); a separate park entrance fee applies |
| **ELEVATION:** | 8,900 feet |
| **RESTRICTIONS:** | *Pets:* On leash only *Fires:* In fire grates only *Alcohol:* At campsites only *Vehicles:* 38 feet *Other:* 7-day stay limit per campsite |

have been known to wander through the campground. (I saw some elk during my visit here.)

Water spigots and comfort stations are spread throughout Rocky Mountain National Park's least busy campground. However, it often fills during the peak season. Timber Creek nears capacity nearly every night from late June to early August. You can generally find a campsite until late in the day Sunday through Thursday. Sites are usually gone by noon on Friday and Saturday. Finding a campsite in the off-season is no problem, though campground roads are not snowplowed.

If you haven't driven Trail Ridge Road, drive it. It is a rite of passage for first-time park visitors. Campers also like to see the wildlife, fish, and hike the area trails. The Never Summer Ranch Trail leaves from the lower part of the campground. It is a mere 0.5-mile walk to this early-era guest ranch. The buildings and grounds have been preserved by the park. Interpretive rangers are on site there in the summer.

The Green Mountain Loop is a popular day hike for Timber Creek campers. It starts down US 34. See Big Meadow and the ruins of a pioneer cabin on this 8-mile tramp. The much shorter River Trail Loop starts down by the Kawuneeche Visitor Center. It runs along the Colorado River and offers views of the Never Summer Mountains above. The path to Timber Lake presents good scenery and is a 10-mile round-trip hike. There are many other trails in the area. The ranger on duty at the campground can steer you on a hike to meet your abilities and desires.

The Colorado River offers fair fishing for brook, brown, rainbow, and cutthroat trout. But serious fishers will head down to the Arapaho National Recreation Area by Grand Lake. The fish are bigger, and the lake is stocked regularly.

Back at the campground, ranger programs are held every night during the summer from mid-June to Labor Day. But mostly campers at Timber Creek will be seen piddling around their campsites. It's called relaxing and having a good time.

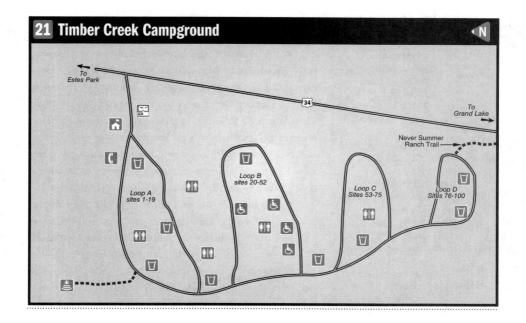

## 21 Timber Creek Campground

To Estes Park

34

To Grand Lake

Never Summer Ranch Trail

Loop B
sites 20-52

Loop A
sites 1-19

Loop C
Sites 53-75

Loop D
Sites 76-100

## GETTING THERE

From Grand Lake, head north on US 34 for 10 miles and Timber Creek Campground will be on your left.

## GPS COORDINATES

| | |
|---|---|
| LATITUDE | N 40° 22' 44.9" |
| LONGITUDE | W 105° 51' 5.6" |

> *Weston Pass is one of the nicer Forest Service campgrounds in Colorado.*

**N**AMED AFTER THE SCENIC BREAK IN the Mosquito Range, Weston Pass is an often-bypassed campground adjacent to an often-bypassed wilderness. I wonder why, since the neatness, cleanliness, and lack of overuse of the campground were evident immediately upon arrival. One look at the mountains of the Buffalo Peaks Wilderness will make you wonder why you didn't get here sooner. The answer lies partly in what surrounds the area—several other, more popular wildernesses and campgrounds lie between the Buffalo Peaks and the major metropolitan areas of the state.

I prefer smaller campgrounds; they are usually a little more out of the way (read: fewer big rigs) and seem to bring out the neighborliness in your fellow tent campers. Weston Pass has only 14 campsites in an area that I've seen fit twice that many at other campgrounds. The campsites are large and spaced very far apart beneath a forest of lodgepole pine that is supported by other evergreens and a few straggling aspen. The ground cover is mostly smaller trees and assorted rocks and boulders. Landscaping timbers and short concrete posts have been tastefully laid out to keep cars and camping areas distinct. This is part of what gives Weston Pass a certain orderliness not always found at other Forest Service campgrounds.

The South Fork of the South Platte River and a low ridge dividing this creek from Rich Creek surround the campground. Head along the main drive and admire the size of the campsites set back in the woods several feet from their respective parking areas. Notice the Ridgeview Trail splitting off between two campsites. The seven sites on the main drive give way to a loop road that swings near the South Fork. The loop offers secluded campsites that drop down toward the clearly audible creek. As the loop swings around, one campsite, 11, is actually a walk-in tent site farther up the creek, away from everyone else. A few more of those large

## RATINGS

**Beauty:** ✿ ✿ ✿
**Privacy:** ✿ ✿ ✿ ✿
**Spaciousness:** ✿ ✿ ✿ ✿
**Quiet:** ✿ ✿ ✿ ✿
**Security:** ✿ ✿ ✿
**Cleanliness:** ✿ ✿ ✿ ✿ ✿

campsites are banked against the low, rocky ridge that shades the campground in the late afternoon.

The well is out by the main road just before you bridge the South Fork. Two vault toilets conveniently serve Weston Pass. This quiet campground rarely fills, except on holidays.

For your evening leg-stretcher, take the Ridgeview Trail 1 mile to an overlook on the point between the drainages of Rich Creek and South Fork. Take note that this trail also connects you to the Rich Creek Trail, which dives into the heart of the Buffalo Peaks Wilderness. The forests here, from piñon-juniper on the lower western slopes to the bristlecone pines of the highlands, are thick with both trees and wildlife, from bighorn sheep to beaver. This area is decidedly lacking in the human species compared to other wildernesses this close to Denver and Colorado Springs.

One of the better day hikes in the Pike National Forest takes off near Weston Pass Campground. Make an 11-mile loop by taking Rich Creek Trail up to Buffalo Meadows and picking up the Rough and Tumbling Trail back down. The Buffalo Peaks Wilderness is also an excellent place to build up your peak-bagging skills. Though they are not fourteeners, East and West Buffalo Peaks exceed 13,000 feet and have definite tree lines that you pass on the way to sizable rock faces to scale with little difficulty. Take the Rough and Tumbling Trail beyond Buffalo Meadows to the headwaters of Rough and Tumbling Creek, then ascend to the pass where the Rough and Tumbling Trail starts to descend. Veer east first to West Buffalo Peak, then East Buffalo Peak. Return to the Rough and Tumbling Trail and backtrack to the campground. This makes a very long day hike, so leave early in the morning for this adventure.

If you don't feel like walking to a view, make the drive up to 11,921-foot Weston Pass. Here, you can look north at a seemingly endless range of peaks. You can also stay down low and fish your way around the South Fork or other waters in the wilderness. Or you can enjoy the subtle, relaxing beauty of the Weston Pass Campground. Pass those other places by for a chance to enjoy the Weston Pass area.

## KEY INFORMATION

| | |
|---|---|
| **ADDRESS:** | Weston Pass Campground South Park Ranger District 320 US 285 Fairplay, CO 80440 |
| **OPERATED BY:** | USDA Forest Service, Pike and San Isabel National Forests, Cimarron and Comanche National Grasslands |
| **INFORMATION:** | (719) 836-2031; www.fs.fed.us |
| **OPEN:** | May–early October |
| **SITES:** | 14 |
| **EACH SITE:** | Picnic table, fire grate |
| **ASSIGNMENT:** | First come, first served; no reservations |
| **REGISTRATION:** | Self-registration on site |
| **FACILITIES:** | Hand-pump well, vault toilets |
| **PARKING:** | At campsites only |
| **FEE:** | $14 per night |
| **ELEVATION:** | 10,200 feet |
| **RESTRICTIONS:** | *Pets:* On leash only *Fires:* In fire grates only *Alcohol:* At campsites only *Vehicles:* 25 feet *Other:* 14-day stay limit |

## GETTING THERE

From the ranger station in Fairplay, drive south on US 285 for 5 miles to CR 5 (Weston Pass Road). Continue on CR 5 until it merges with CR 22 at 7 miles. The campground will be on your left 4 miles ahead on CR 22.

## GPS COORDINATES

**LATITUDE** N 39° 4' 19.9"
**LONGITUDE** W 106° 7' 47"

# NORTHWEST **COLORADO**

**L**ET'S SEE . . . MOUNTAIN biking, canyon hiking, trout fishing, scenic drives, Indian petroglyphs, mining ghost towns, canoeing the Gunnison River . . . all accessible from a free campground made for tent campers that happens to be one of the best in the state. This is Dominguez Canyon. Bureau of Land Management (BLM) campgrounds are generally less known to the public than national-park and national-forest campgrounds. Once you find this little gem, you will be making return trips.

Drop off the Uncompahgre Plateau a bit and descend into Dominguez Canyon. Deep red cliffs are behind you. Below you, bordering Big Dominguez Creek, is a dense forest of large cottonwoods, complemented by thickets of willow and alder, making for a very green scene. Across the canyon, sage gives way to ponderosa pine and Douglas fir intermingling with piñon and juniper.

The air cools down as you approach the clear, chattering creek. Off to your right is a fenced-in grassy area below the cottonwoods. On the far side of a wood fence, three picnic tables lie along the cool waters and offer creekside picnicking. The deep shade and chilled air along the creek create a great escape from the heat of the summer sun in the Colorado River Valley. Farther on, just across the shallow ford of Big Dominguez Creek, lies a single site in the very thick of the cottonwoods. This campsite is for privacy lovers.

Just upstream from this secluded campsite is a small footbridge connecting both sides of the campground. The entrance road fords the creek, and to your right is a small meadow and parking area. An attractive log fence guards more campsites. The cottonwoods here are smaller, still providing ample shade but letting campers enjoy the views around them. Small openings in the fence allow campers to access sites on the far side,

> *Enjoy both the red canyons and green forests of the Uncompahgre Plateau from Dominquez.*

## RATINGS

Beauty: ☆ ☆ ☆ ☆
Privacy: ☆ ☆ ☆
Spaciousness: ☆ ☆ ☆ ☆
Quiet: ☆ ☆ ☆ ☆
Security: ☆ ☆ ☆
Cleanliness: ☆ ☆ ☆

| | |
|---|---|
| **ADDRESS:** | Big Dominguez Campground 2815 H Road Grand Junction, CO 81506 |
| **OPERATED BY:** | Bureau of Land Management |
| **INFORMATION:** | (970) 244-3000; co.blm.gov |
| **OPEN:** | Mid-May– mid-October |
| **SITES:** | 9 |
| **EACH SITE:** | Picnic table, fire ring |
| **ASSIGNMENT:** | First come, first served; no reservations |
| **REGISTRATION:** | No registration |
| **FACILITIES:** | Vault toilets (no water) |
| **PARKING:** | At tent camping parking areas |
| **FEE:** | None |
| **ELEVATION:** | 7,500 feet |
| **RESTRICTIONS:** | *Pets:* On leash only *Fires:* In fire rings only *Alcohol:* At camp- sites only *Vehicles:* None *Other:* 14-day stay limit |

which allows for tent-only camping. The brush rises high enough to make for good campsite privacy.

Three of the first five campsites have two picnic tables each, allowing for larger parties. One campsite is far back in the woods and looks over a mesa that comes to a point above Big Dominguez Creek and an unnamed tributary.

Two other parties joined me on my stay. The small campground rarely fills, so make your plans and come on up. There is no water provided, though springwater from a pipe is located on the entrance road just above the campground. You could also use the water from Big Dominguez Creek and treat it. Two vault toilets have been put in on both sides of the creek.

The campground is perched on the edge of the 70,000-acre Big Dominguez Wilderness Study Area. The BLM expects this area ultimately to become a full-fledged wilderness. One look and you'll agree that it should be preserved.

A good way to get that look is on the Big Dominguez Trail, which starts at the campground. You can head down the canyon and enumerate reasons for preservation. On the lower part of the canyon are Indian petroglyphs; the best way to access the cliff drawings is from Cactus Park. Watch for the sign for Cactus Park on Colorado 141 as you head for the campground, then take the trail toward Triangle Mesa and take the right split down to the Big Dominguez Creek and the petroglyphs. You can also follow the Smith Point Trail up Dominguez Canyon from the campground.

If you like fishing small creeks for trout as much as I do, you'll love Big Dominguez Creek. Take the Big Dominguez Trail down the canyon and simply drop into the creek drainage, then work your way up—secretively I might add—and cast with small spinners. Rainbow trout will positively attack your lure. If you want to ride in the water instead of walking through it, check with outfitters in Whitewater and Grand Junction. The nearby Gunnison River offers some decent canoeing that is more of a relaxed float than a hair-raising whitewater ride.

Mountain bikers take note that the heart of the 140-mile Tabeguache Trail passes right through this campground. You can take the trail up to the plateau or drop

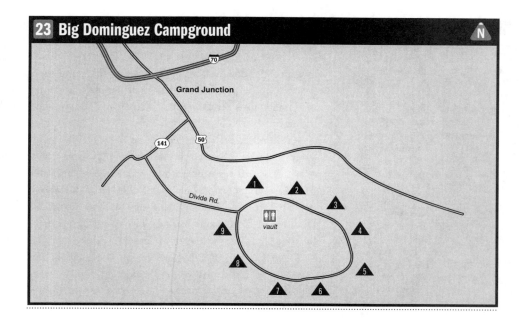

down toward Cactus Park. Send for a map of the Tabeguache Trail from the BLM office in Grand Junction.

Auto tourists will want to return to CO 141 and drive farther up Unaweep Canyon toward Gateway. In the mountains east of Gateway, many old mining sites and miners' shacks are on BLM lands. Again, inquire at the BLM office for details; you'll like what they have to offer in this part of the state.

## GETTING THERE

From Grand Junction, drive southeast on US 50 for 10 miles to CO 141 and the town of Whitewater. Turn right on CO 141 and follow it for 11.5 miles to Divide Road. Turn left on Divide Road and follow it for 5 miles to a fork in the road. Turn left at the fork. There is a sign and arrow saying BIG DOMINGUEZ RESOURCE CONSERVATION AREA. Follow this road 5 miles to Big Dominguez Campground.

## GPS COORDINATES

| | |
|---|---|
| LATITUDE | N 38° 44' 51.9" |
| LONGITUDE | W 108° 33' 41" |

> *Cold Springs is both the grandstand and springboard for enjoying the eastern Flat Tops Wilderness.*

**D**O YOU LIKE CAMPING NEAR A bubbling cascade? Do you like camping near a mountain pond? Do you like camping by a spectacular mountain view? Would you like to enjoy all three of these features and also be next to Colorado's second-largest protected wilderness? Relish all of the above at Cold Springs Campground.

Now, this place isn't perfect, but Cold Springs is an earthly delight. Here, you can leave your tent, fish and hike all day, then return to your little scenic mountain heaven.

All right, let's get to the bad part. It is a little closer to the road than is truly ideal. The campsites could stand to be a little more level. And the campground as a whole is pretty broken in, but other than that, it's great.

Turn into the short campground drive and pass the first campsite on your left, in an open meadow with the best of alpine views. Snow-covered Flat Top Mountain lies across the Bear River, which rushes from Stillwater Reservoir above. Behind you, tree-covered slopes rise to mountain lakes. There is a good view down the valley of Bear River as well.

Cross over a small stream, then enter the small loop road. To your right is the mountain pond. Above it, on the hill, are two other streams noisily dropping over rocks into the pond. The second campsite lies in an open meadow next to the pond and the first stream. This is the largest and most popular campsite. The third campsite is close to the pond as well. It offers all views, but no shade.

The fourth campsite is closest to the cascades and has some shade-providing spruce. The fifth campsite is set off in a forested corner of the campground beside a stream of its own. This is the shadiest and most private campsite. An outhouse lies in the center of the loop and a water spigot is close to all campers in this small campground.

## RATINGS

Beauty: ✪ ✪ ✪ ✪
Privacy: ✪ ✪
Spaciousness: ✪ ✪ ✪
Quiet: ✪ ✪ ✪
Security: ✪ ✪ ✪
Cleanliness: ✪ ✪ ✪ ✪

If Cold Springs is full—with only five sites it may very well be on summer weekends—try Horseshoe Campground just a little way back down Bear River Road. It has seven campsites and is more forested than Cold Springs; consequently, it doesn't have the inspiring views. Cold Springs offers car-free access to the recreational opportunities of the Bear River corridor.

The Flat Tops Wilderness is all around you: cliffs towering over alpine tundra and subalpine terrain, where spruce-fir forests give way to more than 110 fish-filled lakes and ponds. Another 100 miles of streams flow through this angler's fantasyland. Just a 5-minute jaunt up the road from Cold Springs is a major trailhead, Stillwater, leading into the Flat Tops.

To survey your kingdom for a day, take the North Derby Trail, #1122. Cross the Stillwater Dam to a large park, then climb into the wooded highlands through a burned area, coming to an 11,200-foot pass after about 2 miles. Turn left at the pass, leaving the maintained trail, and stay on the divide, rising to the peak of Flat Top Mountain at mile 4. There is a rock pile at the 12,354-foot summit. Look down and see if you can see your friends or spot your tent back at the campsite. You can also stay on the maintained trail and come to Hooper and Keepner Lakes at 3 miles. These are great fishing lakes.

Bear River Trail, #1120, leaves Stillwater Reservoir and goes west into the wilderness. Pass Mosquito Lake at mile 1.5, a scenic yet dubious destination, then climb toward the high country. Once up high, you can go along the Flat Tops in either direction or drop down toward Trappers Lake. The high-country trails are fairly level, for scenic, mild hiking.

East Fork Trail, #1119, splits off Bear River Trail and heads north into some superb vistas. Pass Little Causeway Lake at mile 1.2, then climb up toward the Devils Causeway, a side destination from the East Fork Trail. This is a narrow stretch (4 feet wide) of the Flat Top plateau that drops 1,500 feet in either direction. On the main trail you will come to many small lakes and, finally, Causeway Lake at 5 miles. Anglers, be sure to bring your rods.

## KEY INFORMATION

| | |
|---|---|
| **ADDRESS:** | Cold Springs Campground Yampa Ranger District P.O. Box 7, 300 Roselawn Avenue Yampa, CO 80483 |
| **OPERATED BY:** | USDA Forest Service, Medicine Bow–Routt National Forests, Thunder Basin National Grassland |
| **INFORMATION:** | (970) 638-4516; www.fs.fed.us |
| **OPEN:** | Memorial Day–September 30 |
| **SITES:** | 5 |
| **EACH SITE:** | Picnic table, fire grate |
| **ASSIGNMENT:** | First come, first served; no reservations |
| **REGISTRATION:** | Self-registration on site |
| **FACILITIES:** | Water spigot, vault toilets, trash collection |
| **PARKING:** | At campsites only |
| **FEE:** | $10 per night |
| **ELEVATION:** | 10,200 feet |
| **RESTRICTIONS:** | *Pets:* On leash only *Fires:* In fire grates only *Alcohol:* At campsites only *Vehicles:* 22 feet *Other:* 14-day stay limit |

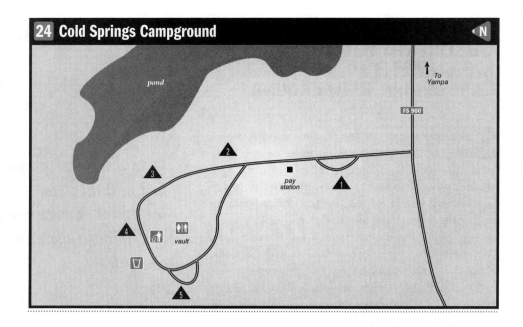

## GETTING THERE

From Yampa, drive southwest on CR 7 for 17 miles as it turns into FS 900. Proceed on FS 900 for about 10 miles. Cold Springs will be on your right.

## GPS COORDINATES

Latitude N 40° 1' 38.3"
Longitude W 107° 7' 29"

For those who want hike-free fishing, there are three reservoirs for fishing in the Bear River Corridor. The closest is Stillwater; Yampa and Yamcola Reservoirs are downstream. In between these reservoirs flows the Bear River. Anglers can be seen bank-fishing the lakes and walking the meadows of Bear River. All these waters are stocked.

Limited supplies can be bought back down in Yampa. When you come to Cold Springs, expect to be busy—the great view at the campground will inspire you to be a part of the scenery.

S OME FOLKS JUST GO FOR IT when they see something. In 1907, Jim Otto came to the canyon country southwest of Grand Junction and deemed it the most beautiful place he had ever seen. He thought it worthy to be a national park; he developed trails single-handedly among the forests and rock sculptures while simultaneously promoting the land with a few converts from Grand Junction. Four years later, Colorado National Monument was established. Jim's devotion to the park persisted until 1927, when he relinquished his $1-per-month job as park caretaker.

> *Deep canyons, red rock, and natural stone sculptures characterize this unique Colorado spectacle.*

What foresight he had in protecting such a colorful landscape! Now, you can enjoy it too. Saddlehorn Campground is near many park features and hosts a few features of its own. After climbing out of the valley below, veer left around the Saddlehorn (it really does look like the horn of a saddle) and enter the campground. A forest of juniper and piñon emerge from the rust-red soil. Occasional rocks emerge from the fiery dirt among the sage. The whole campground has a slight slope toward the cliffs of the Colorado Plateau, which drop off into the Grand Valley of the Colorado River. Across the valley are the East Tavaputs Plateau and the Grand Mesa. The views are striking.

The campground water spigots are tastefully piped into native stone that adds a little extra touch to Saddlehorn. The junipers here are bushy; they provide decent campsite privacy, but the noonday sun will beat you down in midsummer. Be forewarned, from mid-May until early July, small gnats rule this area and can drive you buggy.

Loop A has 20 sites that offer great views into the valley. Several of the sites are screened from the loop road. Loop B is very similar to Loop A and has some very private sites and great views. The lights of Grand Junction shine down below after dark.

## RATINGS

Beauty: ✰ ✰ ✰
Privacy: ✰ ✰ ✰
Spaciousness: ✰ ✰ ✰
Quiet: ✰ ✰ ✰ ✰
Security: ✰ ✰ ✰ ✰
Cleanliness: ✰ ✰ ✰ ✰

**ADDRESS:** Colorado National
Monument:
Saddlehorn
Campground
Fruita, CO 81521

**OPERATED BY:** National Park
Service

**INFORMATION:** (970) 858-3617;
nps.gov/colm

**OPEN:** Loop A all year,
Loop B April–mid-
October, Loop C
when necessary;
no water in winter

**SITES:** 80

**EACH SITE:** Picnic table,
stand-up grill

**ASSIGNMENT:** First come,
first served;
no reservations

**REGISTRATION:** Self-registration
on site

**FACILITIES:** Water spigots,
flush toilets

**PARKING:** At campsites only

**FEE:** $20 per night, plus
$10 entrance fee

**ELEVATION:** 5,800 feet

**RESTRICTIONS:** *Pets:* On leash only
*Fires:* No wood
fires, charcoal fires
in grills only
*Alcohol:* At camp-
sites only
*Vehicles:* None
*Other:* 14-day
stay limit

Loop C is part of the original campground built in the 1930s. The campsites are a little smaller than what we are accustomed to today. It offers views of the valley and into the monument, but Loop C is only open if the other loops are full, which normally occurs during Memorial Day weekend only. Otherwise you can bank on getting a campsite here.

The best time to visit Colorado National Monument, on the advice of a longtime park ranger, is mid-September to mid-November. The weather has cooled, the bugs are long gone, and the hiking is great. You can actually walk from your tent to some of the best day hikes in the park. Window Rock Trail makes a short loop and offers fantastic views. The Canyon Rim Trail travels on the edge of Wedding Canyon for more views. And views are what this monument is all about. Springtime attracts locals for wildflower viewing.

Another ranger recommendation is the Ottos Trail. It drops down toward the Pipe Organ and overlooks the depths of Monument Canyon. If you are here during summer, use the middle of the day to make the 23-mile scenic drive from one end of the park to the other. There are numerous overlooks—you will wear your brakes out stopping at all the dramatic canyon scenes. Road bikers also enjoy pedaling the scenic road. The combination of scenery against the backdrop of the plateau and valley country makes for one photo op after another!

There are several longer trails that range from 6 to 8 miles. Monument Canyon Trail enters the heart of the natural rock sculptures. Climbers can be seen scaling Independence Rock. If you are interested in climbing, stop at the park visitor center, where they have a book on climbing routes in the monument. Whether you climb or not, remember to be up high at dark—the sunsets and sunrises here are something to see. Rangers hold interpretive programs on summer weekends.

Colorado National Monument is a destination in its own right. But if you are traveling along I-70, don't just glance up and say you've seen this place. The scenery will surprise you while you look down at the folks who thought it wasn't worth their time.

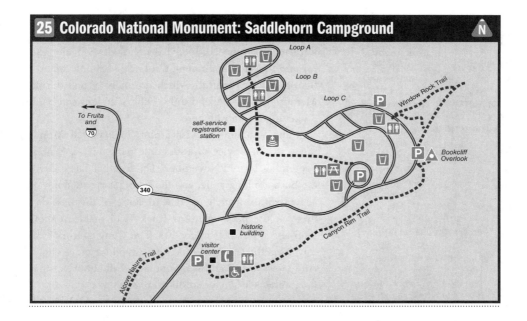

Loop A

Loop B

Loop C

Window Rock Trail

To Fruita and 70

self-service registration station

Bookcliff Overlook

340

historic building

Canyon Rim Trail

visitor center

Alcove Nature Trail

## GETTING THERE

From I-70 in Fruita, head south on CO 340 for 2 miles to the entrance of Colorado National Monument. Proceed into the monument for 5 miles, and Saddlehorn Campground will be on your left.

## GPS COORDINATES

**LATITUDE** N 39° 1'38.9"
**LONGITUDE** W 108° 39' 20"

# 26
# DINOSAUR NATIONAL MONUMENT:
## ECHO PARK CAMPGROUND

> *This is one of the best tent campgrounds in the entire national park system, but you might need an all-wheel-drive vehicle to reach it.*

**T**HE DRIVE DOWN SAND CANYON INTO Echo Park will amaze you. The scenery at Echo Park will stun you. Rough going on the roads is both a blessing and a curse. The thick dust keeps out a lot of campers, and this is one place where you will never, ever, see an RV, unless its driver is demented.

Echo Park lies just below the confluence of the Green and Yampa Rivers. Colorful vertical canyon walls rise from across the river. The grassy meadow of Echo Park leads to another tan, gray, green, and black cliff face enclosing the park. Across the river is the stone sentinel of Steamboat Rock. A dense ribbon of box elder and cottonwood divides much of Echo Park from the river. The opening of Pool Creek Canyon narrows in the distance. More canyon walls and wooded mountains are downriver. The park continues upriver until the Yampa splits off to the right. Words can't begin to describe the true magnificence of Echo Park.

The campground is off to the left, between the river and the meadow as you enter Echo Park. The first campsite is riverside, all by itself; the river access and fee/information booth are past it. Next is a string of four campsites that look over the park from beneath dense, box elder trees. Small paths cut to the river from some of these campsites.

The dirt road continues, then more campsites appear on the riverbank. The picnic tables are lower than the parking spot for these sites. Farther down, the riparian woods break, allowing the next campsites to have views of the Green River and the sheer walls of the canyon beyond. An auto turnaround spot also serves as the parking area for the five walk-in tent campsites that extend upriver.

The first walk-in site sits alone beneath an old cottonwood. The others are a 150-yard walk to a grove of cottonwood and box elder trees that are not as dense

## RATINGS

Beauty: ✿ ✿ ✿ ✿ ✿
Privacy: ✿ ✿ ✿ ✿
Spaciousness: ✿ ✿ ✿ ✿
Quiet: ✿ ✿ ✿ ✿ ✿
Security: ✿ ✿ ✿ ✿ ✿
Cleanliness: ✿ ✿ ✿ ✿

as the vehicle campsites. A water spigot and vault toilet serve these campsites. Other facilities are conveniently situated for all to use, even though the campground is strung over several hundred yards of the river.

You can count on getting a campsite during summer weekdays, but get to Echo Park early on summer weekends. Campsites are nearly always open during spring and fall. However, always call ahead to see if Echo Park is open, as rains can render the road impassable and close the campground.

On your way down Echo Park Road, enjoy the scenery of Sand and Pool Canyons, then stop at Chew Ranch. This site was not developed until the 1900s. The ranch was occupied as late as 1970, when the owner passed on. Other, more primitive ranch sites are also viewable. Next, you will come to a very interesting Indian petroglyph that was scratched high into the Sand Canyon wall. Whispering Cave is farther down. Walk close to it and feel the cool air on a summer day.

The Green River will lure you to its banks, but the swift current can make swimming hazardous. Fishing is negligible for channel catfish, which inhabit the stained waters. The photographic opportunities are numerous. You may also want to bring your camera on some day hikes that leave Echo Park.

The Sand Canyon Route heads up the Green River, then veers right up the Yampa to the first canyon on your right. You can follow the trail for miles up to Yampa Bench Road, but I recommend backtracking—it's less dusty than walking on the road. A good late-afternoon hike is the Mitten Park Route. It follows the Green River downstream, high above the left bank. Hike 1.5 miles to a grassy meadow, Mitten Park. It's another good place to look over Steamboat Rock.

Pats Draw is a quickie canyon-sampler hike. Head back up the road out of the park and veer right just past the second creek ford. This is a short but easy there-and-back walk. You can also start back at the Chew Ranch, then follow the Pool Creek Route up the flow of Pool Creek, though the water course can dry up. It intersects Echo Park Road after 3 miles.

Dinosaur National Monument offers much outside of Echo Park. About 27 miles west of Dinosaur,

## KEY INFORMATION

**ADDRESS:** Dinosaur National Monument: Echo Park Campground 4545 East US 40 Dinosaur, CO 81610-9724

**OPERATED BY:** National Park Service

**INFORMATION:** (970) 374-3000 or (435) 781-7700; nps.gov/dino

**OPEN:** May–September

**SITES:** 22

**EACH SITE:** Picnic table

**ASSIGNMENT:** First come, first served; no reservations

**REGISTRATION:** Self-registration on site

**FACILITIES:** Water spigot, vault toilet

**PARKING:** At campsites only

**FEE:** $8 per night, no fee when water is turned off September–mid-April; park fee also required if you enter at the Dinosaur Quarry area on the Utah side of the park

**ELEVATION:** 5,000 feet

**RESTRICTIONS:** *Pets:* On leash only *Fires:* No wood fires allowed, only charcoal fires in fire pans *Alcohol:* At campsites only *Vehicles:* No RVs or trailers; all-wheel-drive and high-clearance vehicles recommended *Other:* 14-day stay limit

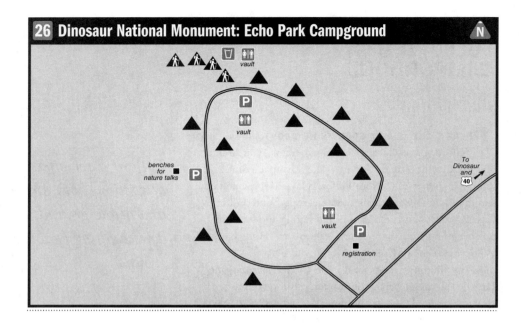

## GETTING THERE

From Dinosaur, head east on US 40 for 1.5 miles to the entrance for Dinosaur National Monument. Turn left on Harpers Corner Scenic Drive and follow it for 23 miles to Echo Park Road. Follow Echo Park Road for 8 dusty miles, then veer right at the signed turn for Echo Park. Follow this road for 5 miles to Echo Park Campground.

Colorado, in the state of Utah, is the Dinosaur Quarry Visitor Center Museum that is overlaid on the fossilized bones of the dinosaurs that made this place a park. Unfortunately this museum, in Jensen, Utah, was closed indefinitely due to significant life, health, and safety issues. However, exhibits, film, fossil displays, ranger-led programs, and information are available in the outdoor visitor center near the park entrance in Jensen, Utah. Harpers Corner Scenic Drive offers a worthy auto tour. Some awe-inspiring views are at the end of day hikes that spur off the scenic drive. Commercial outfitters offer rafting opportunities into the deep canyons of the monument as well. It is impossible to resist telling your friends about this place.

## GPS COORDINATES

**LATITUDE** N 40° 31' 30.5"
**LONGITUDE** W 108° 59' 1.4"

# FULFORD CAVE CAMPGROUND

**T**HERE'S ONE REALLY GOOD THING ABOUT staying at Fulford Cave Campground: if it rains, you aren't necessarily tent bound. You can take advantage of rainy time as a chance to explore Fulford Cave itself, which is less than a mile from this intimate campground. Fulford Cave Campground is in an unusual setting and has other trails leading into the western side of the Holy Cross Wilderness, one of Colorado's best wild places.

The hilltop campground is on the left flank of the East Brush Creek Valley, in a scattered forest of aspen, spruce, and fir. Directly up the watershed is Craig Peak. Below you is the meadow of Yeoman Park. Off to your right, a few hundred feet down a steep rockslide, is East Brush Creek. Just behind the campground is a beaver pond. Off to your left are the trailhead to Fulford Cave and the other trails leading into the Holy Cross Wilderness.

As the forest road dead-ends, the campground is straight ahead and the Fulford Cave Trailhead parking is off to your left. A small spur road splits to the right, where the first three campsites lie. The first one is right on the edge of the drop into East Brush Creek. Be careful after dark if you camp here. The other two sites are by themselves and out of view over a little knob; they offer the most in campsite privacy.

The other four campsites are on a little loop road just as you pull up. One site is in the center of the loop, along with the vault toilet. Two water spigots are available at this diminutive campground. No self-respecting RV or pop-up camper would try to fit in these tent-only campsites. The bigger rigs stay just down the road at Yeoman Park Campground, where you should camp if Fulford Cave ever fills (which it rarely does).

Fulford Cave is Colorado's eighth-largest cavern. More than 2,600 square feet of the underground location has been plotted. Inside are big rooms, narrow

> *Fulford Cave offers attractions both above and below ground. The camping is above ground.*

## RATINGS

Beauty: ✰ ✰ ✰
Privacy: ✰ ✰ ✰
Spaciousness: ✰ ✰
Quiet: ✰ ✰ ✰ ✰
Security: ✰ ✰ ✰
Cleanliness: ✰ ✰ ✰

**ADDRESS:** Fulford Cave
Campground
Eagle Ranger
District
P.O. Box 720125
West Fifth Street
Eagle, CO 81631

**OPERATED BY:** USDA Forest Service, White River
National Forest

**INFORMATION:** (970) 328-6388;
fs.usda.gov/
whiteriver

**OPEN:** June–October

**SITES:** 7

**EACH SITE:** Picnic table, fire pit

**ASSIGNMENT:** First come,
first served;
no reservations

**REGISTRATION:** Self-registration
on site

**FACILITIES:** Water spigot, vault
toilet, summer
trash collection

**PARKING:** At campsites only

**FEE:** $8 per night

**ELEVATION:** 9,400 feet

**RESTRICTIONS:** *Pets:* On leash only
*Fires:* In fire pits
only
*Alcohol:* At campsites only
*Vehicles:* 25 feet
*Other:* 14-day
stay limit

crevices, streams, stalagmites, and stalactites. (Harken back to your school days and try to remember which one develops from the top down and which one builds from the bottom up.) Fulford Cave was discovered during the mining boom of the 19th century by a man named Maxwell, who named the cave after the nearby mining town of Fulford. He never found the riches he sought in the cave, but he did leave a timbered entrance and a pit entrance.

The 0.7-mile trail to the cave starts by the gate at the trailhead parking area. Start making your way up the forest on switchbacks, and you'll soon come to the cave. If you do explore inside the cave, the Forest Service recommends you have the following with you: durable and warm clothing, gloves, hard hat, flashlights and head lamps, sturdy boots, and drinking water. A cave map is available at the ranger station in Eagle. Remember, just like on the surface, you are responsible for your own safety in the cave.

Speaking of on the surface, there are two good trails that head into the Holy Cross Wilderness from Fulford Cave. They both lead to 16-acre Lake Charles. The Lake Charles Trail follows East Brush Creek for 4.4 miles before coming to the lake. Mystic Island Lake is a mile farther. Both lakes offer good fishing for cutthroat trout, while East Brush Creek offers fishing for rainbow, brook, and brown trout. I recommend fishing the stream in the meadows and beaver ponds below Fulford Cave.

The Ironedge Trail is a horse and foot trail. It offers many highlights on its 7-mile journey, as the surroundings change from aspen to fir to alpine tundra above the tree line. Along the way are cabins, meadows, and mine sites, interspersed with good views. The last two miles are downhill to Lake Charles. You can combine the Ironedge Trail with the Lake Charles Trail to make an excellent loop hike. For this particular adventure, you don't need a hard hat.

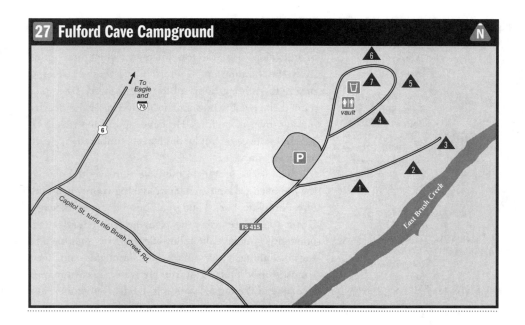

To
Eagle
and
70

6

vault

FS 415

East Brush Creek

Capitol St. turns into Brush Creek Rd.

## GETTING THERE

From the I-70 exit in Eagle, #147, head south on US 6 as it veers right and then makes a sharp left on Capitol Street. Proceed on Capitol Street as it turns into Brush Creek Road for 10 miles and come to FS 415 (East Brush Creek Road). Turn left on FS 415 and follow it 7 miles to Fulford Cave Campground.

## GPS COORDINATES

**LATITUDE** N 39° 29' 29.5"
**LONGITUDE** W 106° 39' 28.0"

# IRISH CANYON CAMPGROUND

> *If you really want to get away from it all, come here. You'll see a whole different side of Colorado.*

**I**RISH **C**ANYON **IS FOR ADVENTUROUS TENT** campers. It is off the beaten path and then some, in the extreme northwest corner of the state on Bureau of Land Management (BLM) land. This is in the Browns Park area, where Butch Cassidy and his gang retreated to safety between heists at the turn of the 20th century. Irish Canyon itself is named for a trio of robbers who lit down the gorge after a hold-up in nearby Rock Springs, Wyoming.

These days you can enjoy the scenery and solitude of Irish Canyon, then venture out to a host of sights, including Indian petroglyphs, Vermillion Falls, Lodore Hall, Browns Park National Wildlife Refuge, the Gates of Lodore, and more.

Irish Canyon is only 100 yards wide as you enter it. High rock walls drop down to sage, grass, and boulder fields. Gnarled old piñon and juniper trees rise along the wall in places. When you come to the campground, the sage gives way to old trees that climb up Cold Spring Mountain. Across the canyon is a sharp, high wall of rock, where small trees cling to precipices. I arrived at Irish Canyon in the afternoon, when the sun burned so brightly into the wall it shone. Later, a full moon rose over the canyon, making it easy to imagine outlaws tending stolen cattle rustled into the gorge.

A teardrop loop enters the forest of old juniper and piñon, above a campsite that overlooks the quiet road traversing the canyon. This site has two tables for larger groups. The second site also overlooks the flat below and the immense wall, but has ample shade.

The campsites farther up the loop are more secluded. The campsite atop the loop is large and is the most private. Three more campsites occupy somewhat leveled areas on the way back down. The picnic table pads have all been leveled, but some tent sites have a slight slope to them. A single vault toilet lies in the wooded interior of the loop for all to use. No water is provided; you must

## RATINGS

Beauty: ✿ ✿ ✿ ✿ ✿
Privacy: ✿ ✿ ✿
Spaciousness: ✿ ✿ ✿
Quiet: ✿ ✿ ✿ ✿
Security: ✿ ✿
Cleanliness: ✿ ✿ ✿

bring your own. Browns Store, 10 miles from the camp and west down CO 318, has water, gas, a phone, and limited supplies. They also rent canoes if you want to float down a quiet section of the Green River.

This is a very isolated camp, but with a road alongside it. So if you worry about leaving your gear unattended, have your adventures, then set up camp and stay there. This area no longer hosts robbers; most passersby are friendly local ranchers, so you needn't be concerned about theft. Nor should you be concerned with Irish Canyon filling up. Campsites are available year-round.

At a place like Irish Canyon, you have to explore and make your own adventures. There are no rangers to tell you what to do or brochures laying everything out. It is wise to contact the BLM office in Craig for information to help you plan exactly what you want to do.

On your way from Maybell, watch for signs leading to local sights and make note of their particular roads. The old coke ovens are near Greystone. The Sand Wash Basin has a herd of wild horses. On the way in, stop at Vermillion Falls. It's a pretty, yet strange, sight—a cascade in such dry land. On old jeep roads, you can also explore by foot or mountain bike Vermillion Creek and its colorful badlands canyon. The Gates of Lodore is the entrance to a magnificent canyon, where the Green River leaves Browns Park and crashes downstream to meet the Yampa River at Dinosaur National Monument. A trail leaves the picnic area at the entrance of the canyon to see some Indian petroglyphs, possibly inscribed by two different tribes on the same rock.

The hiking and mountain biking around Irish Canyon is limited only by your stamina. Marked trails are few, but jeep roads are many. Below the canyon, paths lead up Green Canyon onto Peek-a-boo Ridge and a sweeping view of Browns Park below. Old jeep roads lead up Talamantes Creek farther up the canyon onto Cold Spring Mountain. Unless on foot, stay on the roads.

Drive down to Browns Park National Wildlife Refuge to absorb a little human and natural history. Thousands of birds stop there during spring and fall migration. Elk and deer make this ribbon of green their home during the winter. You can make the 11-mile auto tour of the refuge and see the old Lodore Hall, where

| | |
|---|---|
| **ADDRESS:** | Irish Canyon Campground Little Snake BLM Field Office 455 Emerson Street Craig, CO 81625 |
| **OPERATED BY:** | Bureau of Land Management |
| **INFORMATION:** | (970) 826-5087 or (970) 826-5000; blm.gov |
| **OPEN:** | April 15– November 30 |
| **SITES:** | 6 |
| **EACH SITE:** | Picnic table, steel fire ring |
| **ASSIGNMENT:** | First come, first served; no reservations |
| **REGISTRATION:** | No registration |
| **FACILITIES:** | Vault toilet (bring water) |
| **PARKING:** | At campsites only |
| **FEE:** | No fee |
| **ELEVATION:** | 6,650 feet |
| **RESTRICTIONS:** | *Pets:* On leash only *Fires:* In fire rings only *Alcohol:* At campsites only *Vehicles:* 30 feet, on roads only *Other:* 14-day stay limit |

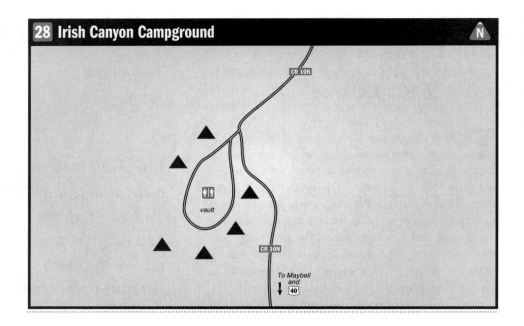

## 28 Irish Canyon Campground

CR 10N

vault

CR 10N

To Maybell
and 40

## GETTING THERE

From Maybell, drive west on US 40 for 0.5 mile, then turn right on CO 318 and follow it for 41 miles to CR 10N. Turn right on CR 10N and follow it 8 miles to Irish Canyon Campground, which will be on your left.

you'll find another petroglyph rock and the Two Bar Ranch. This was the stomping ground of Butch Cassidy. Thanks to the proximity of three states—Colorado, Utah, and Wyoming—ruffians could slip across state lines and out of jurisdiction when lawmen chased them.

I loved this area; finding it was a steal, better than the loot Butch Cassidy and the Wild Bunch were after.

## GPS COORDINATES

LATITUDE N 40° 49' 44.1"
LONGITUDE W 108° 44' 8.5"

# 29 RIFLE FALLS STATE PARK CAMPGROUND

**T**RY THIS ONE ON FOR SIZE: Colorado's favorite year-round waterfall was created from limestone buildup behind an ancient beaver dam, and these are the cliffs we see today. The falls became a 19th-century tourist attraction and were then used as the impetus for Colorado's first hydroelectric plant. The plant was then dismantled and a state park was built around the picturesque site. The state later renovated the park and campground into what we see today. Bet you didn't know beavers could be that constructive.

No matter how the falls came to be—and I am skeptical about that beaver dam story—they are here now and you can delight in them and the lakes of Rifle Gap State Park, Harvey Gap State Park, rock climbing at Rifle Mountain Park, the East Fork Rifle State Fish Hatchery, and more outdoor recreation in the White River National Forest nearby. All this can be enjoyed from your base camp at the pleasing walk-in tent sites set in the riparian lushness of the East Fork Rifle Creek.

Park your car at Rifle Falls and take the Squirrel Trail that runs along East Fork Rifle Creek. The campsites spur off the Squirrel Trail. The first campsite is set beneath tall, narrow leaf cottonwoods and is the only site not along the creek. Continue on and you'll find more sites scattered among the box elder, willow, grass, and cottonwoods of the creek bottom.

All the sites have been renovated and are more appealing than ever. Each campsite is completely separated from the rest; the farther down the path, the more separated the sites become. The stream sends out a constant symphony of whitewater music. The final campsite is mostly surrounded by the creek, and it is the most isolated and one of the best tent sites in the entire state park system.

Thirteen drive-in sites, which cater to RVs, comprise the balance of the campground. These sites have

> *Rifle Falls is the scenic centerpiece of the Rifle Valley. Set up your base camp here and explore the nearby parks and forest land.*

## RATINGS

Beauty: ✰ ✰ ✰ ✰
Privacy: ✰ ✰ ✰ ✰ ✰
Spaciousness: ✰ ✰ ✰ ✰
Quiet: ✰ ✰ ✰
Security: ✰ ✰ ✰ ✰ ✰
Cleanliness: ✰ ✰ ✰ ✰

# KEY INFORMATION

**ADDRESS:** Rifle Falls State Park Campground 00050 Road 219 Rifle, CO 81650

**OPERATED BY:** Colorado State Parks

**INFORMATION:** (970) 625-1607; parks.state.co.us

**OPEN:** All year

**SITES:** 7 walk-in tent sites (Squirrel), 13 drive-in sites (Falls)

**EACH SITE:** Walk-in sites have picnic table, fire grate, tent pad; drive-in sites have picnic table, fire grate, electricity

**ASSIGNMENT:** By reservation or pick an available site on arrival

**REGISTRATION:** (800) 678-CAMP (2267) or (303) 470-1144 in metro Denver, at park entrance, or reserveamerica .com

**FACILITIES:** Water spigot, vault toilets

**PARKING:** At campsites only

**FEE:** $7 Parks Pass plus $16 per night walk-in tent sites Oct.–Apr., $18 per night May–Sept.; $20 per night drive-in sites Oct.–April, $22 per night May–Sept.; an additional $10 fee added to each reservation

**ELEVATION:** 6,500 feet

**RESTRICTIONS:** *Pets:* On leash only *Fires:* In fire grates only *Alcohol:* 3.2% beer only *Vehicles:* None *Other:* 14-day stay limit

been renovated as well and the whole campground has a tidy appearance to it that meets the high standards of Colorado state parks. Water spigots and new vault toilets have been built to serve the area.

If you want to stay here, get a reservation. There is no reason not to make the five-minute phone call to eliminate the horror of a full campground. Get a reservation no matter when you come. This campground is open year-round.

Of course, Rifle Falls will probably be your first visit. Feel the mist as water plunges down three chutes to the pool below. Take the trail to the top of the falls and see the caves that are there too. Another hiking opportunity is the Squirrel Trail, which crosses the creek below the falls and explores the waterside lushness of this valley.

Speaking of water, if you vie for trout in the creek and none bite, head a short way up the valley to the state fish hatchery. They are open for visitation, and at least you can take a look at a trout—actually hundreds of them.

Farther up the valley is Rifle Mountain Park. This is where the rock climbers do their work, scaling the sheer walls of the East Fork Rifle Creek canyon. Even if climbing isn't your thing, check out the free show and admire their bravado. Anglers take note that the creek is stocked up here. Farther up the creek is the White River National Forest. The Three Forks Trail leaves Three Forks Campground and makes a loop up by Coulter Lake back to the Spruce Picnic Area.

Below Rifle Falls is Rifle Gap State Park. Boaters and jet skiers make wakes through the 350-acre impoundment, and there is a swimming beach for those who like their water sports a little slower. The fishing here can be fast or slow, depending on your skill and luck, of course. Harvey Gap State Park offers more aquatic pleasures and is just a few miles away. There is no waterskiing here; you are more likely to see windsurfers cutting a wake. The 160-acre lake has trout and warm-water fish such as smallmouth bass and crappie.

The city of Rifle is nearby for any supplies you might need, so pitch your tent at the falls and enjoy all the sights in this little Colorado valley with a big punch.

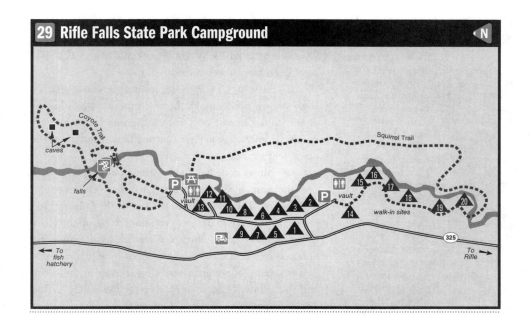

## GETTING THERE

From Rifle, go north on
CO 13 for 3 miles.
Turn right onto CO 325 and
drive 9.8 miles.

## GPS COORDINATES

**LATITUDE** N 39° 39' 46.0"
**LONGITUDE** W 107° 42' 8.7"

> *This is the best tent campground at Trappers Lake, birthplace of the wilderness movement.*

**T**HE **TRAPPERS LAKE AREA IS ONE** of superlative beauty. This beauty is what spawned the wilderness movement as we know it today. In 1919, Forest Service employee Arthur Carhart was surveying the Trappers Lake area in order to lay out a road to and around the lake. He was to plot out some cabin sites on the lake. On seeing the beauty of the forest, water, and cliffs of this high country, he realized this was one place where human works simply couldn't improve on nature. He did complete the survey; however, he let his views be known to his supervisors that some natural places should be set aside in their original state.

This idea of preservation that Carhart started culminated in the Wilderness Act of 1964; today there are more than 3 million acres of wilderness land set aside in Colorado alone. The nearest wilderness, the Flat Tops Wilderness, nearly encircles Trappers Lake. There are several campgrounds in the immediate Trappers Lake area, but Shepherds Rim is the best campground for tent campers.

Shepherds Rim is set in a thick spruce forest that is left intact wherever possible, integrating the campground into the woods. A slight slope has required the Forest Service to erect retaining walls and some steps between the road and the actual camping areas to level the campsites, making them more camper-friendly.

With several small campsites and parking spots, the layout of Shepherds Rim discourages the bigger rigs from camping here, despite the presence of a few drive-through campsites. In general, the abundance of tent pads means a majority of overnight visitors are tent campers.

Enter the long and narrow campground loop, then pass the first drive-through campsite (even though it is drive-through, it also has a tent pad). Most of the campsites are on the outside of the loop, increasing privacy. Short paths connect parking areas to the picnic tables to

## RATINGS

Beauty: ✿ ✿ ✿ ✿
Privacy: ✿ ✿ ✿
Spaciousness: ✿ ✿ ✿
Quiet: ✿ ✿ ✿
Security: ✿ ✿ ✿ ✿ ✿
Cleanliness: ✿ ✿ ✿ ✿

the tent pads. The tent pads are often farther back in the woods, making for better privacy.

The sites at the back of the loop are the most private. There is a special handicapped-accessible site, a double campsite for larger parties, and a campground host to make your stay safe and pleasant. Overall, the Forest Service has upgraded this spot into a well-kept, quality campground that you can use as a base camp to enjoy this area.

Water recreation centers around Trappers Lake, more than 300 acres of picturesque Flat Tops splendor. Cliffs rise above the forest and reflect off the clear, clean tarn, where brook and native cutthroat trout thrive. No motors are allowed here, so bring a paddle along with your canoe to enjoy the peaceful environment. Fishing is by artificial flies and lures only. Possession limit is eight for the nearly pure strain of cutthroats. There is no possession limit on brook trout. Other fishing opportunities are along the North Fork of the White River below Trappers Lake and along Fraser Creek, which feeds Trappers Lake.

You can combine hiking and fishing by using many of the trails that radiate from Trappers Lake into the surrounding Flat Tops Wilderness. The nearest trail to Shepherds Rim is Wall Lake Trail, #1818. It leads up and away steeply from the campgrounds to reach the Flat Tops Plateau after 3 miles. Meadows and forest intermingle here. Wall Lake, 2 miles farther, offers fishing for cutthroat trout.

Carhart Trail, #1815, roughly circles Trappers Lake in a 4.5-mile loop. It parallels the east and north shore of the lake, allowing for angling opportunities, but pulls away from the lake as it crosses Fraser Creek to intersect Wall Lake Trail. Stillwater Lake Trail spurs off Carhart Trail and heads east to Little Trappers Lake and other fishable lakes. It also offers views of the Chinese Wall, an impressive blockade of rock that extends for miles.

Buy all your supplies before coming to Trappers Lake, then plan to stay a while. This body of water and the surrounding Flat Tops are among the best locations in the state—and that is saying a lot.

## KEY INFORMATION

**ADDRESS:** Shepherds Rim Campground Blanco Ranger District 317 East Market Street Meeker, CO 81641

**OPERATED BY:** USDA Forest Service, White River National Forest

**INFORMATION:** (970) 878-4039; fs.usda.gov

**OPEN:** June–mid-October

**SITES:** 15

**EACH SITE:** Picnic table, fire grate, some tent pads

**ASSIGNMENT:** First come, first served; no reservations

**REGISTRATION:** Self-registration on-site

**FACILITIES:** Water spigot, vault toilet

**PARKING:** At campsites only

**FEE:** $18 per night

**ELEVATION:** 9,900 feet

**RESTRICTIONS:** *Pets:* On leash only
*Fires:* In fire grates only
*Alcohol:* At campsites only
*Vehicles:* 36 feet
*Other:* 10-day stay limit; campground borders the wilderness; please obey all wilderness regulations

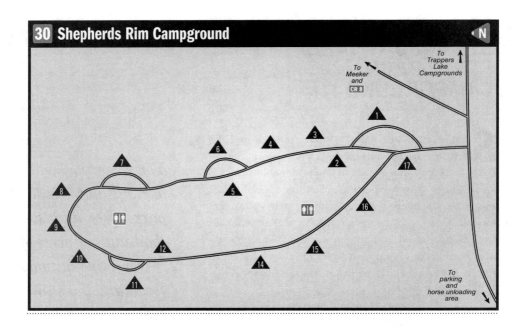

## GETTING THERE

From Meeker, travel east
1 mile on CO 13. Turn right
onto CR 8 to Trappers Lake
Road. Travel 11 miles to the
campgrounds. Turn right.
Shepherds Rim will be
1 mile on the right.

## GPS COORDINATES

**Latitude** N 39° 59' 37.5"
**Longitude** W 107° 14' 29"

# 31
# STEAMBOAT LAKE STATE PARK CAMPGROUND

**S**OME PLACES GET REPUTATIONS. As I scoured the state in search of the best tent campgrounds, Steamboat Lake kept coming up as an unquestionable inclusion for this book. I was expecting something special, and I wasn't disappointed. It started with the new visitor center and ended with the view from the walk-in tent sites from Bridge Island. In between was the town of Steamboat Springs—in my opinion Colorado's most attractive resort—Hahn's Peak, Pearl Lake, and the Mount Zirkel Wilderness.

Don't be turned off by the large number of campsites here. They are divided over two major campgrounds. The tent area is set apart on an island and is the main concern to us tent campers.

Sunrise Vista Campground has 113 sites on the eastern edge of Steamboat Lake. If you are going to stay here, try the Harebell Loop. There will be big rigs here, but this loop nevertheless offers the closest lakeside campsites at Sunrise Vista. The Larkspur Loop is well shaded. The Yarrow Loop also has some lakeside sites, but is dominated by RVs.

The Dutch Hill Campground has 85 campsites. The Wheeler and Baker Loops have electric hookups and are dominated by RVs. Pass the camper services building (with showers, laundry, and so on) near the marina, then arrive at Bridge Island, tent camper's heaven. The first 15 campsites are on a loop beneath lodgepole pines. These are drive-up sites that are a little too crowded for my taste. But they are on the island, and the eight campsites on the outside of the loop are near the water.

But the best is last: On the far side of this loop is the parking area for the tent-only campsites. These last 20 sites occupy the part of the island that juts out farthest into Steamboat Lake. The walk to the sites ranges anywhere from 20 to 200 feet, but the lake and mountain views get better the farther you are from the parking area.

> *You can enjoy not only all that this state park offers but also thousands of acres of surrounding national forest and the resort town of Steamboat Springs.*

## RATINGS

Beauty: ✪ ✪ ✪ ✪
Privacy: ✪ ✪ ✪
Spaciousness: ✪ ✪ ✪ ✪
Quiet: ✪ ✪ ✪
Security: ✪ ✪ ✪ ✪ ✪
Cleanliness: ✪ ✪ ✪ ✪

**ADDRESS:** Steamboat Lake
State Park
Campground
Box 750
Clark, CO 80428

**OPERATED BY:** Colorado State
Parks

**INFORMATION:** (970) 879-3922;
parks.state.co.us/
steamboat

**OPEN:** Mid-May–October

**SITES:** 20 walk-in tent
only, 198 others

**EACH SITE:** Picnic table, fire
grate, tent pad;
55 have electricity

**ASSIGNMENT:** By reservation or
pick an available
site on arrival

**REGISTRATION:** (800) 678-CAMP
(2267) or (303)
470-1144 in metro
Denver, at reserve
america.com, or at
campground booth

**FACILITIES:** Hot showers, flush
and vault toilets,
laundry, phone,
vending machines,
marina store

**PARKING:** At campsites or
walk-in tent camp-
ers parking area

**FEE:** $7 Parks Pass plus
$16–18 per night
walk-in tent sites
or nonelectric
vehicle sites, $20–
22 per night elec-
tric vehicle sites

**ELEVATION:** 8,100 feet

**RESTRICTIONS:** *Pets:* On leash only
*Fires:* In fire grates
*Alcohol:* 3.2% beer
only
*Other:* 14-day
stay limit

The walk-in campsites are situated in wooded areas between fields that are far from one another. A gravel path spurs off the main gravel loop, connecting the campsites. The sites are dispersed so that campers on the interior of the loop have a quality view as well. The southernmost campsites are the best and most isolated. Boaters can actually pull their craft onto the shore of the island and walk to their campsites.

As the loop swings around, the campsites enter heavy lodgepole woods. The view is across to the marina. These are the least desirable, but still good, walk-in sites. Two vault toilets serve the immediate area, though full facilities are nearby at the camper services building.

If you want to stay here, get a reservation, though the tent sites are the last to be filled. This park has a strong following among the locals, which speaks volumes about its quality. Front Range campers make the drive to overnight here, so do out-of-staters. I repeat, make a reservation to secure a campsite.

Steamboat Lake is, naturally, a park attraction. All manner of water sports are enjoyed on the lake. Skiers, anglers, and watercraft enthusiasts use the reservoir. A power zone and a no-wake zone make Steamboat Lake enjoyable for all visitors. The inlets of the lake offer the best fishing for rainbow, brown, arctic grayling, and native cutthroat trout. If you didn't bring your own watercraft, anything from canoes to pontoon boats can be rented at the park marina, where they also have limited supplies.

Nearby Pearl Lake is another scenic jewel of the state park system. It offers trout fishing on a smaller reservoir. The lake is wakeless, so it's a quieter fishing destination.

If you want to get around on foot, first hop in your car and enjoy the Routt National Forest, which nearly encircles Steamboat Lake. Hahn's Peak is a popular hike. The Mount Zirkel Wilderness is east of Steamboat Lake. The Slavonia Trailhead is your best bet for enjoying this glacier-carved highland, where hundreds of alpine lakes dot the landscape. Take the Slavonia Trail up to Gilpin Lake, then loop back down Gold Creek. The Encampment River and North Fork Elk River offer hiking and angling opportunities. A map is sold in the Routt National Forest Visitor Center, which has more than 2,000 square feet of interpretive displays.

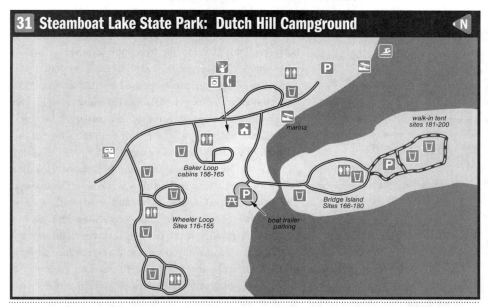

walk-in tent
sites 181-200

marina

Baker Loop
cabins 156-165

Bridge Island
Sites 166-180

Wheeler Loop
Sites 116-155

boat trailer
parking

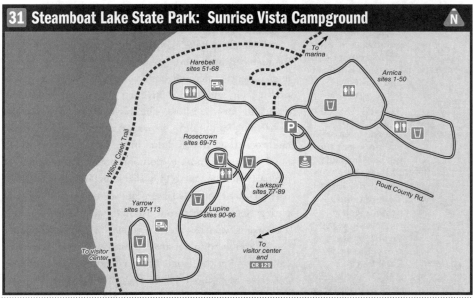

To
marina

Harebell
sites 51-68

Arnica
sites 1-50

Rosecrown
sites 69-75

Willow Creek Trail

Routt County Rd.

Larkspur
sites 77-89

Yarrow
sites 97-113

Lupine
sites 90-96

To visitor
center

To
visitor center
and
CR 129

## GETTING THERE

From Steamboat Springs, drive west on US 40 for 2 miles to CR 129. Turn right on CR 129 and follow it north for 26 miles to Steamboat Lake State Park.

## GPS COORDINATES

**Latitude** N 40° 48' 35.4"
**Longitude** W 106° 58' 5.3"

# 32
# WEIR AND JOHNSON CAMPGROUND

*Lakes are plentiful, and the camping is fine here on top of the Grand Mesa.*

**W**ITH AN AVERAGE ELEVATION OF MORE than 10,000 feet, the Grand Mesa is a cool island of green jutting up from the arid lands of western Colorado. There is a lot of blue up here too, with more than 300 lakes. Several campgrounds are located up here, but my favorite is Weir and Johnson. To begin with, it is off the beaten path at the end of a side road; this makes for less auto traffic. That's important, because when the snow melts up here, recreationists swarm the mesa like mosquitoes to the scenic lakes. And I don't blame them. Once they see how pretty the waters are, rimmed by a spruce-fir forest, punctuated with flowery meadows, they keep coming back year after year. Some come from as far as Tennessee, like the campers I befriended at Weir and Johnson.

This campground also lies between two lakes and has trails leaving the campground to access three more lakes. These lakes are in addition to countless other lakes and the Crag Crest National Scenic Trail that is accessible by auto.

If you have successfully driven to the campground without stopping to wet your fishing line, enter the campground loop. Off to your left are two campsites that are in an area where the Engelmann spruce and subalpine fir have been thinned a bit. As you continue the loop, the western tip of Weir and Johnson Reservoir is off to your right. A third campsite sits across the road from the lake.

As the loop curves, a small cascade rushes downhill past four excellent tent sites down from the loop road beside Sackett Reservoir. You have to carry your gear a bit to reach them, but you are that much closer to the aquamarine water. The next two sites are also down near Sackett Reservoir. The final three campsites are away from the lake, but are heavily shaded. On my early July visit, one campsite was still too snow-covered to use!

## RATINGS

Beauty: ☆ ☆ ☆
Privacy: ☆ ☆ ☆
Spaciousness: ☆ ☆ ☆
Quiet: ☆ ☆ ☆ ☆
Security: ☆ ☆ ☆
Cleanliness: ☆ ☆ ☆

There is a pair of vault toilets for campers. The old pump well is capped—bring your own water and you won't have to take any chances.

You will be taking chances if you try to camp here on July 4 or Labor Day. Weekends can fill, but if you get here by mid–Friday afternoon, you should get a campsite. Campsites are nearly always available during the week.

Trout swim the waters of the two campground reservoirs, and fishing is popular throughout the Grand Mesa, but hike-in lakes often see less fishing pressure. You can walk to Leon Lake. Just cross the Weir and Johnson Dam, hug the shoreline to the right, and cross a small pass to Leon Lake, which is larger than Weir and Johnson. Round Lake and Leon Peak Reservoir are nearby too. Cross the Weir and Johnson Reservoir dam, then bear left when the trail splits.

After seeing all these lakes, I was wishing for my canoe. Bring yours or borrow one; you can really get around to less-fished spots on all these lakes up here, nearly 2 miles high. And there is hardly more scenic paddling in the state. If you bring a motorboat, check the regulations—many lakes are too small for motorized craft and don't allow them.

Hiking "The Crag" is tops for foot travel on the Grand Mesa. The Crag Crest National Scenic Trail is a 6.5-mile path that rides the spine of the mesa and offers views in all directions of far-off mountain ranges. On this inspiring hike, you can see all the lakes lying below you like emerald jewels in the forest. The Crag Crest Connector Trail passes through forest and meadow to complete a 10-mile circuit. You can pick up "The Crag" back on FS 121 near The Crag Crest Campground, which you passed on the way in.

More information can be obtained at the Grand Mesa Visitor Center at the junction of Colorado 65 and FS 121. Supplies can be purchased at a small store a couple of miles east on FS 121 from the visitor center.

## KEY INFORMATION

| | |
|---|---|
| **ADDRESS:** | Weir and Johnson Campground Grand Valley Ranger District 277 Crossroads Boulevard, Suite A Grand Junction, CO 81506 |
| **OPERATED BY:** | USDA Forest Service, Grand Mesa, Uncompahgre, and Gunnison National Forests |
| **INFORMATION:** | (970) 242-8211; fs.usda.gov |
| **OPEN:** | July–September |
| **SITES:** | 12 |
| **EACH SITE:** | Picnic table, fire grate |
| **ASSIGNMENT:** | First come, first served; no reservations |
| **REGISTRATION:** | No registration |
| **FACILITIES:** | Vault toilets |
| **PARKING:** | At campsites only |
| **FEE:** | $12 per night |
| **ELEVATION:** | 10,500 feet |
| **RESTRICTIONS:** | *Pets:* On leash only *Fires:* In fire grates only *Alcohol:* Allowed *Vehicles:* 20 feet *Other:* 14-day stay limit |

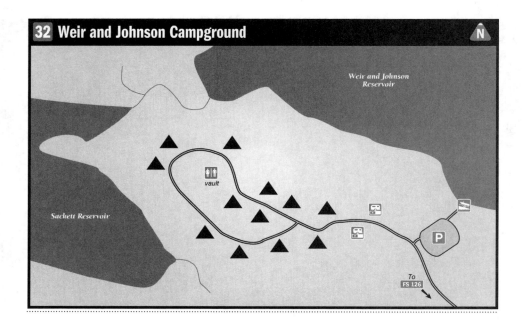

## GETTING THERE

From Cedaredge, head north on CO 65 for 15 miles to FS 121. Turn right on FS 121 and follow it for 9 miles to FS 126. Turn right on FS 126 and follow it 3 miles to the dead end at Weir and Johnson Campground.

## GPS COORDINATES

**LATITUDE** N 39° 4' 0.9"
**LONGITUDE** W 107° 49' 53.0"

SOUTH CENTRAL **COLORADO**

# 33
# ALVARADO CAMPGROUND

**A**LVARADO IS AN ACTIVE PERSON'S CAMPGROUND. On a summer Saturday there will be hikers, bikers, and horseback riders gearing up and heading out on their favorite trails. Several of the trails leave directly from the campground, which is a nice place to return after a day in the scenic Sangre de Cristo Mountains.

Alvarado meets the banner standard set by the Sangre de Cristos. On a slope just into the forest line above the Wet Mountain Valley, Alvarado enjoys a mixture of woodland and meadow, where Douglas fir and ponderosa pines intermingle with aspen. Cottonwood and brush grow thick along Alvarado Creek. Forest density varies with exposure on the three loops. So no matter what your preference for sun or shade, view or privacy, your wishes should be fulfilled, unless it is a weekend holiday, the only time the campground fills.

The first few campsites are in a meadow overlooking the mountains across the valley, then the main road enters a ponderosa grove. The right-hand road, with several nice campsites along it, leads to the Venable Trailhead, which is located at the end of this loop. The main campground road continues upward, with campsites on a rocky slope beneath the pines. Another road splits off to the right into a grove of aspen. It has several campsites that offer much shade and some views of Comanche Mountain, high in the Sangre de Cristos above. The road switchbacks farther up the mountain with more shaded and isolated campsites, then comes to a set of five walk-in, tent-only sites. Here, you park your car and walk a short distance to set up camp. But these sites are on a slope and you may be hard-pressed to find a level place to pitch your tent. However, the entire campground is suitable for tents. This road ends at a turnaround and the Comanche Trailhead.

The final set of campsites are on a side road of their own in a ponderosa grove off the main campground

> *Alvarado is on the eastern slope of the Sangre de Cristo Mountains.*

## RATINGS

Beauty: ✪ ✪ ✪ ✪
Privacy: ✪ ✪ ✪ ✪
Spaciousness: ✪ ✪ ✪
Quiet: ✪ ✪ ✪
Security: ✪ ✪ ✪ ✪
Cleanliness: ✪ ✪ ✪ ✪

## KEY INFORMATION

**ADDRESS:** Alvarado Campground San Carlos Ranger District 3170 East Main Street Cañon City, CO 81212

**OPERATED BY:** USDA Forest Service, Pike and San Isabel National Forests, Cimarron and Comanche National Grasslands

**INFORMATION:** (719) 269-8500; fs.usda.gov

**OPEN:** Memorial Day weekend–mid-Oct.

**SITES:** 47

**EACH SITE:** Picnic table, fire grate

**ASSIGNMENT:** First come, first served for some, reservations for 27 of the sites required

**REGISTRATION:** Self-registration on site, call (877) 444-6777 or visit reserveusa.com

**FACILITIES:** Water spigot, vault toilets, trash pick-up, electricity and phone available at host station

**PARKING:** At campsites only

**FEE:** $17 per night, an additional $9 fee added to each Internet or phone registration

**ELEVATION:** 9,000 feet

**RESTRICTIONS:** *Pets:* On leash only *Fires:* In fire rings only *Alcohol:* At campsites only *Vehicles:* 35 feet *Other:* 14-day stay limit

road. Water spigots and vault toilets are spread throughout the campground, which is very large to have only 47 campsites. Many of the sites are spread quite far apart. A campground host is stationed at the entrance to the campground for your safety.

Hikers, bikers, and horse riders all enjoy the area trails, most of which lead into the far-flung Sangre de Cristo Wilderness. The Comanche Trail heads up along Alvarado Creek to Comanche Lake. The Venable Trail leads up a couple of miles to Venable Falls, then a few more miles to the Venable Lakes areas. Most of these lakes don't thaw out until late June. You can combine the Comanche and Venable Trails and make a strenuous 13-mile loop via Phantom Terrace back to the campground.

If you are looking to stretch your legs but not climb straight uphill, try the Rainbow Trail. It runs 46 miles all the way from south of Alvarado north to Salida. You can use the Rainbow Trail to connect to other trails entering the Sangre de Cristo Wilderness. The Godwin Trail, one watershed north, climbs to alpine lakes. The Cottonwood Trail, one watershed south, climbs along Cottonwood Creek. Any of these bodies of water are suitable for fishing.

You can also drive to within a quarter mile of Hermit Lake, another alpine body of water high in the mountains. Take County Road 160 (Hermit Road) west out of Westcliffe and drive 13 miles to a signed parking area near the lake. Bring your fishing pole.

You can reward yourself after all that exercise with a good meal at the Alpine Lodge, which is located a few steps from the campground. Or you can drive into Westcliffe and take the walking tour of the downtown area. Get your self-guiding brochure at the Tourist Information Center caboose. There is ample food, drink, and supplies here in town.

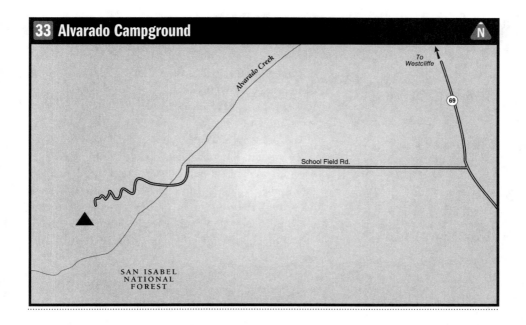

## GETTING THERE

From the courthouse in Westcliffe, drive south on CO 69 for 3 miles to CR 140 (School Field Road). Turn right on CR 140 and follow it for 6 miles to Alvarado Campground.

## GPS COORDINATES

**LATITUDE** N 38° 4' 45.7"
**LONGITUDE** W 105° 34' 4.9"

> *The magnificent Sangre de Cristo Mountains provide a scenic backdrop for Bear Lake.*

**S**NOWY, GRANITE DOMES OF THE SANGRE de Cristo Mountains plunge down to a forest of spruce and fir. This in turn gives way to an open meadow and Bear Lake, where you can enjoy tent camping, in the most southeasterly slice of national-forest land in Colorado. Fishing comes naturally with all the water around, both still and moving. You can move along many trails in the vicinity and make a side trip to the Spanish Peaks, a National Natural Landmark.

The campground is well placed next to the dense forest and mountain meadow above Bear Lake. Along the campground's gravel loop, several wooded campsites are situated to your right with obscured views of Bear Lake. More open sites with occasional stray aspen are in the center of the loop as the road swings around into the grassy meadow. What these campsites lack in privacy they make up in views of Steep Mountain above, the nearby meadow, and a cathedral of peaks beyond. A few campsites on the outside of the loop face into the clearing, which has a stream flowing through it.

The Indian Creek Trailhead starts just beyond campsite 9. The loop road begins to climb into the forest again. Another creek rushes from the high country through the campground to Bear Lake. The next few campsites are in the spur to your right, offering the most in campsite privacy.

This is one of the highest campgrounds around, so bring that extra blanket and expect to find temperatures around, or possibly below, freezing throughout the summer. Be prepared for windy, cool conditions any time at Bear Lake. Stake your tent down extra-taut as well, because the gusts of wind from the peaks above can blow mighty strong. Cover yourself from the penetrating rays of the sun. Experience taught me these lessons the hard way. On my visit I failed to bring enough clothes for the chill, my face got sunburned, my tent was blown

## RATINGS

Beauty: ✿ ✿ ✿ ✿
Privacy: ✿ ✿
Spaciousness: ✿ ✿ ✿
Quiet: ✿ ✿ ✿ ✿
Security: ✿ ✿ ✿ ✿
Cleanliness: ✿ ✿ ✿ ✿

over, and I froze my tail off that night. And I still like this place.

Vault toilets are located at the center of the loop and near the Indian Creek Trailhead. An old-fashioned pump provides water at the height of the campground. For your safety and security a campground host is situated at the beginning of the loop. Bring your supplies, as it is a far piece to the nearest full-service grocery store.

After setting up camp, why not check out Bear Lake? A foot trail circles the deep blue trout-laden water fed by streams from above. Drop in a line or two. No luck? Try Blue Lake. It's a mile by foot or road to the almost equally scenic fishing waters. You'll pass a few other small lakes along the way if you walk. For anglers who prefer moving water, try fishing Cuchara Creek. It winds along Forest Service Road 422, your route up to Bear Lake.

Hikers have two nearby options in addition to Bear and Blue Lakes. Take Indian Creek Trail from the campground north to Bonnet Park or make a loop via Baker and Dodgeton Creeks. Ambitious hikers will want to take the 3.5-mile gut-buster up the old North Fork four-wheel-drive road to Trinchera Peak (13,517 feet). The view will get your heart pumping again. This trek starts near Blue Lake.

Take your camera just south of Bear Lake on Colorado 12 to Cuchara Pass. FS 46 leads from the pass to the Spanish Peaks. These two granite domes are an offshoot of the Sangre de Cristo Mountains and will deliver scenery overload if you head to and beyond 11,000-foot Cordova Pass.

The isolation and long drive with no population base nearby make this a quiet campground, though there may be some site competition on summer holidays. Just come better prepared than I was.

## GETTING THERE

From La Veta, drive south on CO 12 for 13 miles to FS 422. Turn right on FS 422 and follow it for 5 miles to Bear Lake Campground.

## GPS COORDINATES

LATITUDE  N 37° 19' 32.5"
LONGITUDE  W 105° 8' 36.0"

# 35
# GREAT SAND DUNES NATIONAL PARK & PRESERVE: PINYON FLATS CAMPGROUND

**I**T WAS AN INCREDIBLY WINDY DAY as I headed toward the dunes. Dust and sand were blowing across the San Luis Valley. Blanca Peak towered on my right, somewhat clouded by the airborne grit. Later, the Great Sand Dunes appeared, a massive shifting swath of sand, contrasting with the verdant Sangre de Cristo Mountains in the background. The blustery day made it evident how such a peculiar sight could form in the middle of the Rocky Mountains.

Pinyon Flats Campground, located in the Great Sand Dunes National Park and Preserve, impressed me as well. It is set in a juniper-pine forest complemented with a sagebrush and grass understory between the dunes and the high country. There are two long, narrow loops, each with a variety of campsites to suit almost anyone. The Dunes Trail and seasonally flowing Garden Creek bisect the Pinyon Flats.

Loop A is lower and closer to the dunes. A paved road cuts down on dust. Low stone walls level the ground and define boundaries between the 44 campsites. Large rocks keep cars where they are supposed to be. Some campsites are nestled in piñon thickets; others are more open. But the open campsites offer views of the dunes and mountains. Most sites are spacious. As the loop circles back, campsites drop down from the road toward the dunes. These sunny sites offer incredible views of the sands, but they have a more worn and dusty appearance to them.

Loop B parallels Loop A, but is situated on higher, more wooded ground. It has 44 campsites as well and a few cottonwoods growing alongside Garden Creek, breaking up the evergreens. Elaborate rock work keeps the natural areas from being trampled and levels the campsites. Just beyond the Little Medano Trailhead is a set of campsites that offers great views of the contrasting sand dunes and mountains.

> *You can't imagine the sight of America's largest sand dunes perched against the Rocky Mountains. Come see it for yourself.*

## RATINGS

**Beauty:** ☆ ☆ ☆ ☆
**Privacy:** ☆ ☆ ☆
**Spaciousness:** ☆ ☆ ☆
**Quiet:** ☆ ☆ ☆
**Security:** ☆ ☆ ☆ ☆ ☆
**Cleanliness:** ☆ ☆ ☆ ☆ ☆

## KEY INFORMATION

**ADDRESS:** Great Sand Dunes National Park and Preserve: Pinyon Flats Campground 11999 CO 150 Mosca, CO 81146

**OPERATED BY:** National Park Service

**INFORMATION:** (719) 378-2312, nps.gov/grsa; (877) 444-6777, recreation.gov

**OPEN:** All year

**SITES:** 88

**EACH SITE:** Picnic table, fire grate, tent pad

**ASSIGNMENT:** First come, first served and by reservation

**REGISTRATION:** Camping permit required; self-registration on site

**FACILITIES:** Water spigots, flush toilets, community sinks

**PARKING:** At campsites only

**FEE:** $20 per night

**ELEVATION:** 8,200 feet

**RESTRICTIONS:** *Pets:* On leash only
*Fires:* In fire grates only
*Alcohol:* At campsite only
*Vehicles:* 35 feet
*Other:* 6 people maximum per site; 14-day stay limit

Each loop has two comfort stations with flush toilets, drinking water, and sinks for washing your dishes. Between Loop A and Loop B is a small campground store that is open between May and September. It offers typical camp supplies, such as ice, wood, and soda. If you run out of something, buy it here; otherwise, I suggest making a major supply run before you get to the dunes.

Pinyon Flats can fill on summer weekends. It is a little on the busy side during summer weekdays. Grab a reservation and you will be fine. However, from September to May, the campground is quiet and most campsites are available. Late spring and early fall are the best times to visit.

Have you ever climbed a 700-foot sand dune? Here's your chance. Take the half-mile Dunes Trail from the campground down to the dunes and start climbing. The loose sand and deceptive distances make it more challenging than it seems. This is one place where your footprints never last for long. Eighteen miles of more foot-friendly trails lace the park. Head north from the campground on the Little Medano Trail 1.2 miles to a cliff overlooking the dunes. The Pinyon Flats Trail connects the campground with the visitor center. The Wellington Ditch Trail is an easy hike along an old settler's irrigation flow. The high country awaits you on the Mosca Pass Trail.

In the summer, there are ranger-led walks every day and ranger programs every evening. Keep your camera handy at all times. The ever-changing light and dunes combine to present an evolving landscape as you explore the environment. These are the largest sand dunes in North America. The unexpected setting for them makes the Great Sand Dunes experience an eye-opening reward and very worth the stop.

Outside the park is the short walk to Zapata Falls. It is on public land a few miles south of the monument on Colorado 150. You can extend the hike 3 more miles up to alpine Zapata Lake. Nearby San Luis Lakes State Park offers fishing, boating, and wildlife viewing. Thousands of acres of the Sangre de Cristo Wilderness lie east of the dunes. A primitive road skirts the monument and heads into this vast national-forest land.

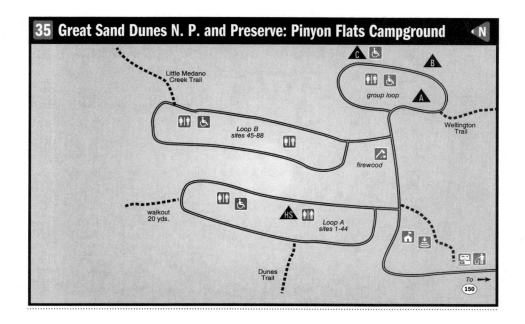

Little Medano
Creek Trail

group loop

Wellington
Trail

Loop B
sites 45-88

firewood

walkout
20 yds.

HS

Loop A
sites 1-44

Dunes
Trail

To →
150

## GETTING THERE

From Blanca, drive west on
US 160 for 5.2 miles to CO
150. Turn right on CO 150
and follow it for 16 miles to
Great Sand Dunes National
Monument.

## GPS COORDINATES

LATITUDE N 37° 44' 46.9"
LONGITUDE W 105° 30' 17"

> *Cool off in the lake country of the San Juan Mountains.*

**S**UMMER COMES LATE HIGH IN THE San Juan Mountains. Mix Lake, at 10,000 feet, enjoys the blessings and curses of a short season. It is blessed with light use and a stunning high-country landscape, but the season is short and the weather can be rough. The campground is integrated into the varied topography and vegetation of the land. Mix Lake is scenic itself, but so are other nearby lakes, Platoro Reservoir, and the rugged South San Juan Wilderness.

After you pass the pay station, the gravel campground road begins to switchback upward toward Mix Lake. As you turn, the first three campsites surprisingly appear on your right in a clearing surrounded by aspen. These sites are fairly close together, but offer good views of the Conejos River valley below. Continue up the mountain and pass campsite 4, all by itself. It has a good view and also offers the most solitude. Campsite 5 is perched on a hill with even better views, but is very close to the road.

Then come to the first loop, set in a mixed bag of brush, rocks, grass, and scattered trees. The campground host resides here. The loop enters a dense conifer stand, with campsites offering nearly complete shade and privacy. The sites in the center of the loop are more open. These sites and those at the end of the loop avail views of the valley below and the mountains above. Nearly all of the 12 campsites are spread far from one another.

The second loop is the highest and closest to Mix Lake. It also offers just about any combination of sun and shade. There are five campsites here. The two sites closest to the short trail to the lake are the most heavily used. There is a water spigot at the beginning of this loop.

Mother Nature did an excellent job of landscaping this campground. The combination of meadows, boulders, trees, and views will satisfy even the pickiest tent camper. There are three vault toilets in this widespread

## RATINGS

Beauty: ✿ ✿ ✿
Privacy: ✿ ✿ ✿ ✿
Spaciousness: ✿ ✿ ✿
Quiet: ✿ ✿ ✿ ✿
Security: ✿ ✿ ✿ ✿
Cleanliness: ✿ ✿ ✿ ✿

campground. One is down the hill by the first three campsites; the other two are in the two main loops.

The long drive and nearby private resorts conspire to make this a quiet campground. Expect to find a site on all but the busiest summer weekends. Supplies can be had in the little village of Platoro just a mile down the hill. Expect to be gouged a bit when you buy them.

There are, however, many good things nearby, like Mix Lake itself. A short trail leaving the upper loop will take you to an overlook. Beyond is the massive Conejos Peak. Dark blue Mix Lake sits waiting below, with rainbow trout ready to match wits with you. Just a mile distant is the much larger Platoro Reservoir. This dammed lake is 700 acres in size and offers rainbow and brown trout. Just up toward Stunner Pass are Lily Lake and Kerr Lake. These are accessible from Forest Service Road 257.

There are three convenient trailheads leading into the remote South San Juan Wilderness. The weathering of volcanic rock over the ages by wind, water, and glaciers has left jagged peaks, alpine lakes, and towering forests. Rugged trails and the lack of 14,000-foot-high mountains keep the crowds away. Two trails enter the wilderness from FS 105. Take Trail 719 for the short but steep climb past Tobacco Lake on the way to Conejos Peak, 13,172 feet of rock offering unspoiled views of the wilderness and beyond. After climbing Conejos Peak you'll be glad it wasn't 14,000 feet. Head up to Bear Lake on Trail 721. Or take a trip to the Three Forks, where the headwaters of the Conejos River come together. This trail, 712, starts beyond Platoros Reservoir. The Continental Divide Trail runs 40 miles through the length of the wilderness. Below the wilderness, the Conejos River is a popular fishing destination itself. The river scenery has been recommended for wild and scenic designation. It is interspersed with private holdings, so be careful about where you wet your line.

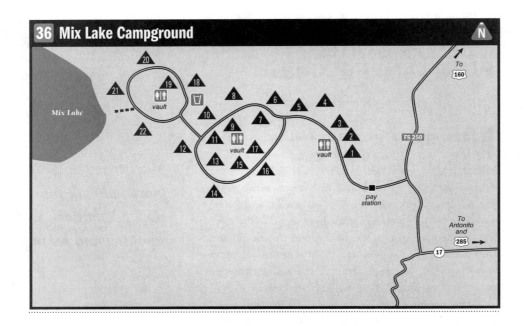

## GETTING THERE

From Antonito drive 22 miles west on CO 17 to FS 250. Turn right on FS 250 for 24 miles to the signed left turn for Mix Lake Campground. Follow this road for 1 mile to Mix Lake Campground.

## GPS COORDINATES

**Latitude** N 37° 21' 29.8"
**Longitude** W 106° 32' 48"

**M**ANY CLAIM MUELLER STATE PARK TO have views and scenery in Colorado second only to Rocky Mountain National Park. While this is debatable, it is evident that Mueller is blessed with a panoramic piece of land. Pikes Peak is in full view to the east, and a long stretch of the Continental Divide lies in sight to the west. The immediate spruce, fir, and aspen slopes, broken with meadows and rock outcrops, serve as the canvas on which a clean, well-kept campground and a complete network of trails make up Mueller State Park.

The commendable upkeep of quality facilities is immediately noticeable when you arrive at Mueller. While riding the smooth, paved road to the immaculate, well-groomed campground, you'll wish all tenting locales could look this nice. The camping area is set in the high country along Revenuers Ridge, with several roads spurring off the main ridge road. The first spur road is Peak View. Here, five campsites are set in woods that look up to Pikes Peak. These sites are usually dominated by RVs and are among 11 total campsites that are open year-round.

The main campground road, divided into two one-way roads, has campsites all along it, including several pull-through sites. Then, Conifer Ridge splits off to the right. True to its name, spruce, fir, and pine cloak its slopes. All types of campers enjoy this area. Farther up Revenuers Ridge on your left is Prospectors Ridge. Here is a 12-site walk-in tent camping area. The woods are thick and campsites are strung out far from one another for more than 100 yards. If you want the maximum in solitude and privacy, pitch your tent here.

More campsites are laid out along the main road as you continue to Turkey Meadow. The meadow is a ten-site, walk-in tent camping area. Pine and fir trees shade most of the campsites, except those on the meadow's edge; no matter where you are, the view of Pikes

> *Mueller is the ideal place to break into Rocky Mountain tent camping and hiking.*

## RATINGS

Beauty: ✿ ✿ ✿ ✿ ✿
Privacy: ✿ ✿ ✿
Spaciousness: ✿ ✿ ✿
Quiet: ✿ ✿ ✿
Security: ✿ ✿ ✿ ✿ ✿
Cleanliness: ✿ ✿ ✿ ✿ ✿

## KEY INFORMATION

Peak is majestic. Feel fortunate if you get one of these campsites.

The campground ends with more campsites and an auto turnaround on Grouse Mountain. The tent camping areas are the best, but there is not a bad site in this well-designed campground. Water spigots and vault toilets are situated throughout Mueller. The showers, flush toilets, and laundry facilities are centrally located in the Camper Services building.

This campground stays booked from June through August. If you want to stay here—and I highly recommend that you do—come during the week, and make reservations no matter what time of year you camp. It is an ideal starter park for camping novices, and veterans will appreciate the extra special touch the state puts on at Mueller.

The same goes for recreation here. The trails are well marked and maintained. There are more than 85 miles of pathways, most open to both bikers and hikers of all skill levels. Some trails are also open to horseback riders. In the backcountry, you can hike to views, open meadows, and old homesteads and mines. There are several ponds in the backcountry for folks to fish. Four-Mile Creek offers stream fishing for trout.

The south end of Mueller has the Four-Mile Day Use Area. This is the trailhead for the popular hike up to Dome Rock. This trek involves several creek crossings. You may see some bighorn sheep from this rock, which rises 800 feet above the valley below.

Park personnel can steer you in the right direction for a trail of your ability. Go to the visitor center for answers to questions and also check out the indoor wildlife habitat there. Rangers lead nature programs during the summer in this wildlife-rich park of 12,000 acres. Mueller State Park can get you on your way to being a Rocky Mountain hiking and camping pro.

Also, while you are in the area, make a side trip to the mining town of Cripple Creek and Victor. The historic mining communities have been revamped, offering a little history and a lot of gaming.

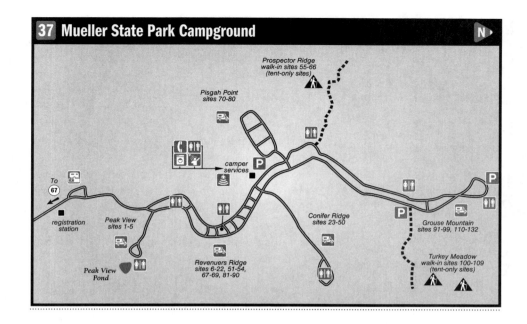

Prospector Ridge
walk-in sites 55-66
(tent-only sites)

Pisgah Point
sites 70-80

camper
services

To
67

registration
station

Peak View
sites 1-5

Peak View
Pond

Revenuers Ridge
sites 6-22, 51-54,
67-69, 81-90

Conifer Ridge
sites 23-50

Grouse Mountain
sites 91-99, 110-132

Turkey Meadow
walk-in sites 100-109
(tent-only sites)

## GETTING THERE

From Woodland Park, drive west on CO 24 for 7 miles to Divide. Then turn left on CO 67 south for 3.5 miles to Mueller State Park, which will be on your right.

## GPS COORDINATES

**Latitude** N 38° 54' 5.9"
**Longitude** W 105° 9' 43"

# 38
# NORTH CRESTONE CREEK CAMPGROUND

> *North Crestone offers creekside camping in a riparian forest perched against the Sangre de Cristo Mountains.*

**N**ORTH CRESTONE IS ONE OF THE best campgrounds in southwestern Colorado. Most other campgrounds are in a woodland with two or three tree types. Here, along North Crestone Creek, grows an abundance of tree types, especially by Rocky Mountain standards. The campground's location in a forest transition zone along a well-watered valley produces this biodiversity. Cottonwoods, piñon pine, juniper, Douglas fir, maple, alder, and aspen conspire to form a dense forest, where campsites are nestled into nooks and crannies between streamside boulders.

Being in the foothills of the Sangre de Cristo Mountains contributes to making this a desirable place to tent camp. Craggy, barren, snow-covered peaks, alpine lakes, far-reaching views of the San Luis Valley and mountains beyond make the hiking some of the most scenic in the state. The upper reaches of these highlands are protected wilderness.

The campground begins just after you enter the Rio Grande National Forest. On your left is a rocky, tree-studded canyon wall. To your right is the crashing Crestone Creek, shaded by all those wonderful trees. A heavy understory of younger trees and alder screens you from everyone else.

The first set of campsites are set into the woods. The camper parking spots are along the two-way road. At each site, the picnic tables and fire grates are located a short walk from the parking spots closer to the creek. A vault toilet and pump well serve these campsites.

The next set of campsites are farther up the road by a good 100 yards. These campsites are notched into flat areas among the boulders and trees wherever they can fit. There are a couple of sites that offer some sun, but expect to be in the shade most of the time in this valley environment.

## RATINGS

Beauty: ✿ ✿ ✿ ✿ ✿
Privacy: ✿ ✿ ✿ ✿ ✿
Spaciousness: ✿ ✿ ✿
Quiet: ✿ ✿ ✿ ✿
Security: ✿ ✿ ✿
Cleanliness: ✿ ✿ ✿ ✿

The final set of two campsites is located just before the end of the road and trailhead parking. One campsite is across the road from the creek—it's the only one that isn't directly next to North Crestone Creek. A vault toilet and pump well are also up here. A vehicle turnaround and the mountains lie beyond the last campsites.

This is a popular weekend campground, being so beautiful and having so few sites. The upside of having only 13 sites is that even when it's busy, it doesn't seem crowded. But if you want to camp here on a weekend, try to get here on Friday night or early Saturday morning. You won't regret losing a little sleep to camp at North Crestone.

The Sangre de Cristo Wilderness is just a walk away from your tent. The North Crestone Creek Trail leaves the upper end of the campground, heads up, and connects to other trails in the wilderness, enabling trips to the high country. Venable Pass is 5 miles distant, as is North Crestone Lake. The trails here are well marked and maintained. You can fish the creek, which tumbles as waterfalls much of the distance, or North Crestone Lake, where the fishing is said to be good. Wildlife-viewing possibilities include seeing bighorn sheep and bears. Speaking of bears, they are known to slip into the campground during lean years, so store your food properly.

Campers sometimes walk the mile to the hamlet of Crestone. Here they have a small general store, a tavern, and an eatery. The living is nice and slow here. No tourist traps, just nice people. While you are down there, check out a few more hiking opportunities.

If you take the road past the post office in tiny Crestone and follow it 2 miles up, you will come to the South Crestone and Willow Lake Trails. South Crestone climbs a few miles to South Crestone Lake. Willow Lake Trail leads 3 miles to Willow Lake and Willow Falls. This whole country is very photographer-friendly. I believe the Sangre de Cristos are the most scenic mountains in Colorado. Come here and rate them for yourself.

## KEY INFORMATION

**ADDRESS:** North Crestone Creek Campground Saguache Ranger District 46525 CO 114 Saguache, CO 81149

**OPERATED BY:** USDA Forest Service, Rio Grande National Forest

**INFORMATION:** (719) 655-2547; fs.usda.gov

**OPEN:** Mid-May–October

**SITES:** 13

**EACH SITE:** Picnic table, fire ring

**ASSIGNMENT:** First come, first served; no reservations

**REGISTRATION:** Self-registration on site

**FACILITIES:** Pump well water, vault toilets, trash pick-up

**PARKING:** At campsites only

**FEE:** $9 per night

**ELEVATION:** 8,300 feet

**RESTRICTIONS:** *Pets:* On leash only *Fires:* In fire grates only *Alcohol:* At campsites only *Vehicles:* 25 feet *Other:* 14-day stay limit

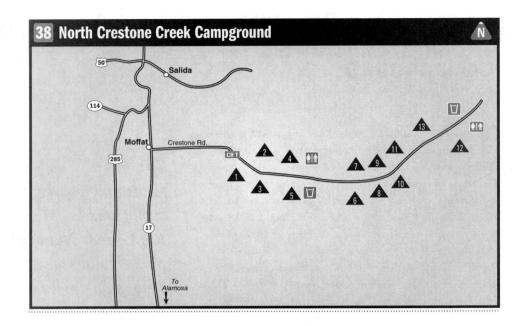

## GETTING THERE

From Moffat, drive east on CR T (Crestone Road) for 13 miles to the hamlet of Crestone. Follow CR T for 1.2 miles until it turns into FS 950. North Crestone will be on your right.

## GPS COORDINATES

**LATITUDE** N 38° 0' 57.8"
**LONGITUDE** W 105° 41' 21"

# 39
# TRUJILLO MEADOWS CAMPGROUND

**T**RUJILLO MEADOWS EXUDES A HIGH-MOUNTAIN AURA from its perch near Cumbres Pass and the New Mexico state line. Thick stands of conifers yield to open clearings of grass where cool breezes make summer wildflowers sway back and forth against the backdrop of the San Juan Mountains. The campground is spread wide over the montane setting, standing at 10,000 feet, making the 49-site getaway a much more intimate spot. Trujillo Meadows Reservoir is an attractive mountain impoundment that anglers and canoers can enjoy. The historic Cumbres and Toltec Railroad chugs through Cumbres Pass, offering scenic tours between Chama, New Mexico, and Antonito, Colorado. Possibly the most remote and rugged wilderness in Colorado, the South San Juan Wilderness is only a few miles away. There, hikers have an opportunity to get back to the Colorado that the Indians knew.

> *This is one of the more scenic and well-kept campgrounds in the Rio Grande National Forest, with much to see and do nearby.*

Leave the well-maintained FS 118 and enter Trujillo Meadows. Pass the campground host, located at the entrance for your safety. The upper loop, starting with site 1, is much more open. The campsites are set among forest and meadow, giving campers many site, shade, and privacy options. A sunny site may be a good choice on a cool, early summer day.

The second loop, starting with campsite 16, has many tent-camping sites but also has pull-through sites that will attract the big rigs. Whoever camps here will enjoy good mountain views, as much of this loop is in open meadowland with only occasional tree cover. Another small loop spurs off this loop but is often closed unless the campground is full.

Keep forward and enter the lower portion of the campground. Here you will find campsites 25 through 49 in an ultradense spruce and fir woodland, which gives off those evergreen aromas that I associate with the high country. This loop slopes off toward a small canyon lying

## RATINGS

Beauty: ✩ ✩ ✩ ✩
Privacy: ✩ ✩ ✩ ✩
Spaciousness: ✩ ✩ ✩ ✩
Quiet: ✩ ✩ ✩
Security: ✩ ✩ ✩ ✩ ✩
Cleanliness: ✩ ✩ ✩ ✩

# KEY INFORMATION

**ADDRESS:** Trujillo Meadows
Campground
Conejos Peak
Ranger District
15571 CR T-5
La Jara, CO 81140

**OPERATED BY:** USDA Forest
Service, Rio
Grande National
Forest

**INFORMATION:** (719) 274-8971;
fs.usda.gov

**OPEN:** Memorial Day–
Labor Day

**SITES:** 49

**EACH SITE:** Picnic table,
fire grate

**ASSIGNMENT:** First come,
first served;
no reservations

**REGISTRATION:** On site

**FACILITIES:** Water spigots,
vault toilet

**PARKING:** At campsites only

**FEE:** $18 per night

**ELEVATION:** 10,100 feet

**RESTRICTIONS:** *Pets:* On leash only
*Fires:* In fire grates
only
*Alcohol:* At camp-
sites only
*Vehicles:* 25 feet
*Other:* 14-day
stay limit

off to the right. The sites here are fairly close together, but the crowded forest eliminates privacy issues, actually making this the campground's most private loop.

Save your walking for the wilderness trails here, as bathrooms and water spigots are spread evenly through-out the campground. Expect Trujillo Meadows to fill on holidays and weekends in the later summer. Get your supplies in the surrounding lowlands; stores are very scarce in the San Juans.

Trujillo Meadow Reservoir lies just a short distance from the campground. Anglers can cast their line for trout. If you bring a boat, keep your large motors home, as this reservoir is wakeless. A canoe or kayak would be a better watercraft choice.

For hikers, the South San Juan Wilderness is as wild as Colorado gets and has more than 180 miles of trails to tramp. The last known grizzly bear in the state was killed here in 1979; many folks think if there are grizzlies left anywhere in Colorado, it will be here in the South San Juans. This place is rugged. Pick up the Continental Divide Trail at Cumbres Pass and head north into the South San Juan Wilderness. For closer wilderness access, take FS 1C to the upper Los Piños River Trailhead (you passed it on FS 118 to the campground). Take Trail 736 and enter an alpine land of jagged mountains and spar-kling lakes. Other trails spur off Colorado 17 on the way up from Antonito. Take Trail 733 up to Red Lake.

For a less sweaty way to see the scenery, take the Cumbres and Toltec Scenic Railroad. Ride in an open-air car, pulled by a coal-burning locomotive, and get an eyeful of mountainous border country. It was originally built in the 1870s to access the mining fields of the Silverton area. The Cumbres and Toltec Railroad is now listed on the National Register of Historic Places. So climb aboard, and let those old-time engines do all the work.

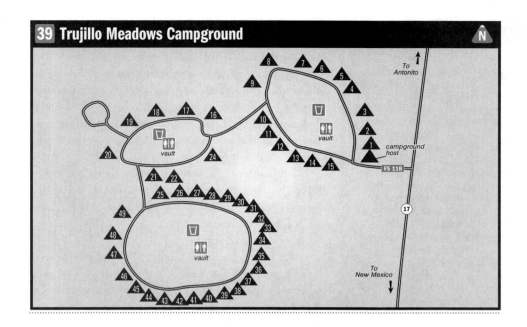

## GETTING THERE

From Antonito drive 37 miles west on CO 17 to FS 118. Turn right on FS 118 and follow it 2 miles to Trujillo Meadows Campground, which will be on your right.

## GPS COORDINATES

**LATITUDE** N 37° 2' 48.3"
**LONGITUDE** W 106° 26' 55"

# SOUTHWEST **COLORADO**

# 40
# BLACK CANYON OF THE GUNNISON NATIONAL PARK:
## NORTH RIM CAMPGROUND

**Y**OU WON'T BELIEVE WHAT A DEEP and narrow gorge the Black Canyon is until you actually see it. There are many places to access the gorge, but the North Rim is the best. It is the most quiet and boasts the better campground in the park, set on the rim's edge in an ancient piñon-juniper forest. Instead of looking up at snowy mountains—your typical Colorado view—you will be looking down into a nearly 2,000-foot-deep canyon. Views can be had by hiking or by a scenic drive. You can hike along the rim or drop down into the gorge itself, where the fishing is great along a stretch of Colorado's Gold Medal Waters. The best climbing in the state can be done here at "The Black," as it's known in the climbing world.

Make your drive from Crawford and slightly descend to the canyon along Grizzly Gulch. Turn right, pass the ranger station, and come to the North Rim Campground. Enter the loop and the piñon-juniper forest, which is complemented with Gambel oak and the bird-attracting serviceberry. As you look for a campsite, note the gnarled trees here. Some are more than 700 years old! It is a rare opportunity indeed to camp among such ancient trees.

The campground lies on a fair slope heading down toward the canyon. The smaller gorge of SOB Draw (which is short for what you think it is) wraps around the campground. Campsites are on both sides of the road beneath the old trees, which offer the ideal amount of sun and shade. The understory is primarily dirt, which can make for a dusty campsite. Overall, the campsites are on the small side, which discourages nearly all but tent campers, especially after big rig drivers see how the old trees crowd the road. They just turn right around. A vault toilet and water spigot are in the center of the small campground. Be advised that the water may not be turned on early or late in the camping season.

> *The North Rim Campground is a rock climber's mecca. If you don't climb, come here anyway; there are other ways to enjoy the gorgeous scenery.*

## RATINGS

Beauty: ✩ ✩ ✩ ✩
Privacy: ✩ ✩ ✩
Spaciousness: ✩ ✩ ✩
Quiet: ✩ ✩ ✩ ✩
Security: ✩ ✩ ✩ ✩ ✩
Cleanliness: ✩ ✩ ✩ ✩

## KEY INFORMATION

**ADDRESS:** North Rim Campground 102 Elk Creek Gunnison, CO 81230

**OPERATED BY:** National Park Service

**INFORMATION:** (970) 641-2337; nps.gov/blca; (877) 444-6777, recreation.gov

**OPEN:** Mid-May–mid-Oct.

**SITES:** 13

**EACH SITE:** Picnic table, fire grate

**ASSIGNMENT:** First come, first served and by reservation

**REGISTRATION:** Self-registration on site

**FACILITIES:** Water spigot, vault toilet

**PARKING:** At campsites only

**FEE:** $12 per night; $7 park pass per vehicle, $9 campsite reservation fee

**ELEVATION:** 7,700 feet

**RESTRICTIONS:** *Pets:* On leash only *Fires:* In fire grates only *Alcohol:* At campsites only *Vehicles:* 26 feet *Other:* 14-day stay limit

At the end of the loop is the Chasm View Trail. During my visit with a friendly ranger, he raved about this trail. I just had to hike it first thing. Even after the hype, the view into the gorge was simply unbelievable. It is so narrow and deep! The Gunnison River emits its roar, but it is fairly faint up here. There are old trees on the Chasm View Trail too. It made me want to hit the other views in the park.

The North Vista Trail leaves from the ranger station. The path goes along the North Rim of the Gunnison to a high point on a nearby ridge. There are views into SOB Draw. But the highlight is the side trip to Exclamation Point. And as the ranger stated, "They call it Exclamation Point for a reason." Some of the best views of the inner canyon are found here.

So you want to make the challenging descent to, and more challenging ascent from, the canyon floor? There are three ways in from the North Rim. The SOB Draw Route starts near the campground. It is two hours down and four hours up the 2-mile route. Watch for the poison ivy growing thick along the way. Long Draw is a mile-long drop that starts near the Balanced Rock Overlook; beware of poison ivy growing 5 feet high here. Slide Draw is very steep and starts near the Kneeling Camel View. Anglers in search of the big trout can brave the poison ivy and test the lesser-fished waters.

There are views along the 5-mile gravel road where you can tour the North Rim by car. Simply leave the campground and keep driving along the rim. Be very careful—the views are quite distracting. At the end of this road is the Deadhorse Trail. This 2.5-mile path traces an old road past springs and provides views into Deadhorse Gulch and the main canyon.

The ranger on duty near the campground is often a climbing ranger. The ranger has a route book for climbers to consult and will assist you in choosing routes. Inexperienced climbers should first go with other climbers or stick to the trails. All climbers and backcountry visitors must obtain a free backcountry permit at the ranger station.

The Black Canyon of the Gunnison is a unique physical feature of Colorado and is a must-see for both natives and tourists.

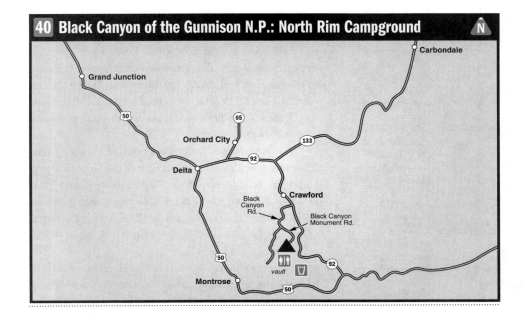

Carbondale

Grand Junction

50

65

Orchard City

133

92

Delta

Black Canyon Rd.

Crawford

Black Canyon Monument Rd.

50

vault

92

Montrose

50

## GETTING THERE

From Crawford, drive south on CO 92 for 3 miles to Black Canyon Road. Turn right on Black Canyon Road and follow it as it twists and turns through the countryside for 6 miles to Black Canyon Monument Road. Turn left on Black Canyon Monument Road and follow it for 5 more miles to the monument. Once at the monument, turn right at the first intersection to access the North Rim Campground, just a short distance away.

## GPS COORDINATES

**LATITUDE** N 38° 47' 14.3"
**LONGITUDE** W 107° 50' 15"

*Burro Bridge is next to the Lizard Head Wilderness, which encompasses the high peaks of the San Miguel Mountains.*

**Y**OU'VE HEARD THE SAYING BEFORE ABOUT real estate—the three most important things are location, location, location. Location is indeed the best thing about Burro Bridge. The site of the small campground is the head of a meadow, fringed in woodland on a perch above the West Dolores River. It meets the expectations of high-country beauty you've come to expect in Colorado's national-forest campgrounds. However, the nearby Lizard Head Wilderness exceeds the beauty expected from the state's wilderness areas. The state's westernmost fourteener and views of the arid, red rock country to the west are two highlights of this wilderness. And proximity to the Lizard Head makes Burro Bridge a tent camper's choice campground. Tent campers with horses are welcome here too.

The 14 campsites are strung along a two-way gravel road with a vehicle turnaround at the end. Aspen and spruce are the primary forest components. The understory is grass, flowers, and young aspen. To your left are the meadow and a rising mountain of solid aspen. To your right is the small canyon of the West Dolores River. An attractive log fence borders the campground along the edge of the precipice that drops down into the West Dolores River. (The Forest Service doesn't want you to fall into the river on a midnight bathroom run.)

The first campsite is nestled in a shade-lending spruce coppice. The next two are by the canyon, but are more open and each has a shade tree near the picnic table. Farther down, a few sites are away from the river in the sunny meadow. This affords little shade but good views of the surrounding mountains.

The road climbs gently up along the meadow, passing the vault toilets for each gender, a pump well, and a small horse corral. Campsites continue on both sides of the road, sunny sites on the left and shadier sites on the right. There is a campsite surrounded by young aspen in the middle of the vehicle turnaround.

## RATINGS

Beauty: ✿ ✿ ✿
Privacy: ✿ ✿ ✿
Spaciousness: ✿ ✿ ✿ ✿ ✿
Quiet: ✿ ✿ ✿ ✿
Security: ✿ ✿ ✿
Cleanliness: ✿ ✿ ✿

The last three sites on the outer auto turnaround are beneath a thick stand of spruce and are very shady. The last campsite is set far from the road and is Burro Bridge's most private site. Overall, the large distance between campsites makes privacy less of an issue and abundant site spaciousness the norm.

With so many campgrounds in the area and being farther from the main roads, Burro Bridge receives light use. You may have it all to yourself on a weekday. Weekends may see a few other tent and horse campers, but expect to find a campsite on all but the major summer holidays.

Though it is not the highest peak, the 400-foot spire at its top makes Lizard Head the most conspicuous mountain in the wilderness. It is not scalable except by expert climbers. There are three fourteeners (Colorado-speak for 14,000-foot or higher mountains) in the Lizard Head. Alpine lakes, waterfalls, and deserted mines complement the high mountains.

Your ticket to all this is the Navajo Lake Trail, which starts a mile above Burro Bridge. The trail crosses the West Dolores, passes two sets of falls, then comes to Navajo Lake. Much of this hiking will be at or above the timber line, so bring clothing for foul weather. A good loop hike uses Navajo Lake Trail then returns to the road above Burro Bridge on the Kilpacker Trail. A little of this hike will be on a forest road.

A good view of the peaks of Lizard Head can be seen while driving over to Colorado 145 to Lizard Head Pass. The historic Rio Grande Southern Railroad wound through this pass. Start a high-country hike from Lizard Head Pass to the spire of Lizard Head on the Lizard Head Trail.

The Calico Trail is also nearby Burro Bridge. Use Forest Service Road 471 to make this 17-mile network of trails any length you like. Mountain bikers should take note of the Stoner Mesa area. This and the Taylor Mesa area offer 150 square miles of high-country forest for hikers, bikers, horse riders, and four-wheel-drive vehicles. Set up camp at Burro Bridge, get out your San Juan National Forest map, and begin exploring.

## KEY INFORMATION

**ADDRESS:** Burro Bridge Campground Mancos-Dolores Ranger District 100 North Sixth Street Dolores, CO 81323

**OPERATED BY:** USDA Forest Service, San Juan National Forest

**INFORMATION:** (970) 882-7296; fs.usda.gov

**OPEN:** June–September

**SITES:** 14

**EACH SITE:** Picnic table, fire ring

**ASSIGNMENT:** First come, first served; no reservations

**REGISTRATION:** Self-registration on site

**FACILITIES:** Pump well water, vault toilets, trash pick-up, horse corrals ($5 per day)

**PARKING:** At campsites only

**FEE:** $14 per night

**ELEVATION:** 9,000 feet

**RESTRICTIONS:** *Pets:* On leash only
*Fires:* In fire rings only
*Alcohol:* At campsites only
*Vehicles:* 35 feet
*Other:* 14-day stay limit

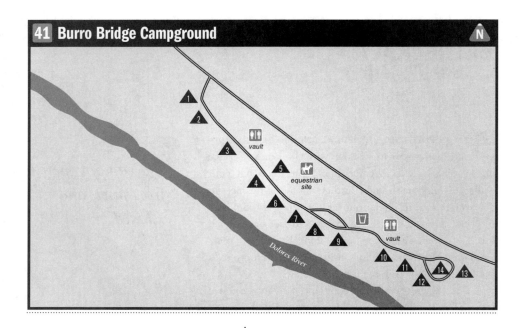

## GETTING THERE

From Dolores, drive north on CO 145 for 13 miles, then turn left on FS 535 (West Dolores Road). Follow FS 535 for 25 miles to Burro Bridge Campground, which will be on your right.

## GPS COORDINATES

**LATITUDE** N 37° 47' 6.3"
**LONGITUDE** W 108° 3' 56"

**A**S YOU PULL INTO CATHEDRAL AND look for a camp-site, you begin to wonder why the Forest Service doesn't charge you to camp here. Then you pat your wallet, dismiss the thought, and go about the business of choosing a spot to pitch your tent. And there are plenty of good campsites in this campground, set in a mixed forest of aspen and blue spruce along Embargo Creek. Cathedral Rock and the La Garita Mountains loom over the locale from across the creek.

The 29 campsites are split about evenly on two loops. The left-hand loop is higher up along the creek. In fact, the upper part of this loop lies astride the confluence of Embargo and Cathedral Creeks. A small clearing lies in the lower center of the loop, as campsites are strung along the heavily wooded banks of Embargo Creek. The forest here is so dense that many of the campsites receive almost no sunlight at all. Others are more open as the loop enters a pocket of old aspens. Then the loop turns back downstream and comes to the clearing again. There is a little rock, Engelmann spruce, and ground juniper thrown into the forest mix. Vault toilets are located at each end of the loop for easy access.

The right-hand loop drops down along Embargo Creek. The woods are denser throughout this loop with very few sunny sites. Judging by the vegetation growing on some of the vehicle pull-in areas on the upper part of the loop, these sites receive very little use. The lower sites along the creek, though, get taken first (and taken they were on my visit). Three of the campsites were occupied by families that had been coming here for years; the trip to Cathedral was a sort of summer pilgrimage for them. They lauded the attributes of Cathedral until they found out it was going to be included in a campground guidebook, then about-faced and made Cathedral sound like a mosquito-infested hole. Well, it is neither heaven nor hell for tent campers, but it is a

> *The camping here is free, quiet, and relaxed.*

## RATINGS

Beauty: ✿ ✿ ✿ ✿
Privacy: ✿ ✿ ✿
Spaciousness: ✿ ✿ ✿
Quiet: ✿ ✿ ✿ ✿
Security: ✿ ✿
Cleanliness: ✿ ✿ ✿

## KEY INFORMATION

**ADDRESS:** Cathedral Campground Divide Ranger District 13308 West US 160 Del Norte, CO 81132

**OPERATED BY:** USDA Forest Service, Rio Grande National Forest

**INFORMATION:** (719) 657-3321; fs.usda.gov

**OPEN:** Mid-April–mid-December

**SITES:** 29

**EACH SITE:** Picnic table, fire grate

**ASSIGNMENT:** First come, first served; no reservations

**REGISTRATION:** No registration

**FACILITIES:** Bring your own water; vault toilets

**PARKING:** At campsites only

**FEE:** No fee

**ELEVATION:** 9,400 feet

**RESTRICTIONS:** *Pets:* On leash only
*Fires:* In fire grates only
*Alcohol:* At campsites only
*Vehicles:* 35 feet
*Other:* 14-day stay limit

nice slice of forest in which to relax and escape the trials of modern life. Cathedral is rarely more than half full—usually less than that—and it is very quiet. It fills maybe one or two weekends per season. The woods provide ample privacy, and the sites are average in size. It does have a worn-in look, like an old, comfortable shoe. This shoe will fit most tent campers.

Relaxing and getting away from it all are at the top of the list here. But if you get tent fever, there are some good hiking trails that leave right from the campground, and other trails are nearby. Cathedral Creek Trail starts near campsite 1 and leads up Cathedral Creek to the Cathedral Rock. In early summer, wildflowers line the trail. Later in the summer you'll be eating strawberries and gooseberries. There are many crossings of the creek, eventually passing a waterfall on the way up to the jagged cliffs of Cathedral Rock.

Embargo Creek Trail leaves the upper loop and heads toward Mesa Mountain along Embargo Creek. Views open up a few miles from the campground. Fremont Camp Trail starts up Forest Service Road 640 a short piece above the campground. Here is where explorer John Fremont and his men spent a long and deadly winter.

Both Cathedral and Embargo Creeks offer excellent trout fishing near the campground. Fly-fishing is easier below the campground in the lower elevations along Embargo Creek, where the forest is more open. But if you want to go for the big ones, head down to the Rio Grande. Many portions of the river are Colorado gold-medal fishing waters, which are catch-and-release areas, allowing the trout to grow larger. Rafting is also a popular way to enjoy the Rio Grande. The rapids are generally Class II and III. Outfitters are stationed in both South Fork and Del Norte.

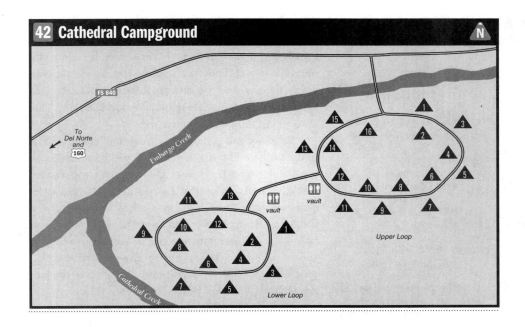

## GETTING THERE

From Del Norte, head west on US 160 for 9 miles to Embargo Creek Road. Turn right on Embargo Creek Road and follow the signs for Cathedral Campground 15 miles distant on FS 650 then FS 640. Cathedral Campground will be on your right.

## GPS COORDINATES

| | |
|---|---|
| **LATITUDE** | N 37° 49' 24.1" |
| **LONGITUDE** | W 106° 36' 16" |

*The view is so good here that the Forest Service should charge a fee instead of letting you camp free.*

**T**HE SETTING AT LOST LAKE CAMPGROUND is classic. A shimmering jewel of water is perched high in the mountains with a forested backdrop, from which snowy, granite twin peaks rise majestically. Most of the campsites have views of this inspiring sight, as if the Kebler Pass Road wasn't scenic enough on the way up to Lost Lake. Rising out of the West Elk Wilderness, East Beckwith and West Beckwith Mountains form twin sentinels over Lost Lake Slough, the body of water beside which you camp. The actual Lost Lake is farther up in the mountains, less than a mile distant.

Not only do you have some of the most scenic tent camping in Colorado, you are also within a mile of two wilderness areas: the West Elk and the Raggeds Wilderness to your north, which were those pointed peaks off to your left as you drove up. So if you get bored with relaxing and fishing at Lost Lake, there are nearly 300 miles of trails between the two wilderness areas on which to exhaust yourself.

When you finally make it to Lost Lake Slough, veer left; to your right are some Forest Service–owned cabins. The main drive runs along the lake, and the first two campsites are large and have popular lake views. Next are a few campsites that are directly lakeside on some less-than-level terrain. The view from here, however, may be worth a sloping night in the tent.

Beyond this, come to the campground drive, which leads away from the lake onto a hill wooded with conifers. The shade is welcome here on those relentless summer days, and the privacy is enhanced by the trees; however, your view of the mountains and lake is obstructed. A small meadow slopes off the drive at the turnaround. You pass one campsite in the center of the turnaround that is convenient to the vault toilet and one more campsite downslope in the woods opposite the lake. This last campsite is generally the last to be taken.

## RATINGS

Beauty: ✿ ✿ ✿ ✿ ✿
Privacy: ✿ ✿ ✿
Spaciousness: ✿ ✿ ✿
Quiet: ✿ ✿ ✿ ✿
Security: ✿ ✿ ✿
Cleanliness: ✿ ✿ ✿

In the summer, Lost Lake will fill up on weekends. Earlier in the season, the weather can be chancy here. As always, call ahead before making the long drive to camp here or anywhere. The campground opening is dependent on the snow up here. The Forest Service will open the campground as soon as the road is open. If the campground is open, you should have no trouble finding a campsite on a weekday.

The serrated, prominent spires of the Ruby Range give the Raggeds Wilderness its name. Aspens and conifers grace the lower, wooded slopes. Trails lead into this land off Kebler Pass Road, both before and after the turnoff to Lost Lake Campground. On your way up, you passed the trailhead for Trail 836, which leads down Trout Creek. To enjoy the higher alpine country, drive toward Kebler Pass and head north on Trail 830, which passes a few lakes as it runs parallel to the Ruby Range.

A short walk away from the campgrounds is the Beckwith Pass Trail, which heads south into the 17,600-acre West Elk Wilderness. Your hike leads south to Beckwith Pass, which isn't usually passable until mid-July. It is a little more than 2 miles to the pass. From there, you can split left to the Cliff Creek Trail, which is actually just before the pass, or continue into the heart of the West Elk. Allow yourself ample time to return before dark.

Closer to home is Three Lakes Trail, which departs from the campground. It offers a 3-mile loop hike that extends to the timber line and passes the actual Lost Lake and Dollar Lake. The views of the Beckwiths are better than the fishing on these upper lakes. The fishing at Lost Lake Slough is considerably better to begin with, and is periodically restocked. You can either bank fish or get onto the lake in any hand-propelled craft. No motors are allowed.

## KEY INFORMATION

**ADDRESS:** Lost Lake Campground Paonia Ranger District P.O. Box 1030 North Rio Grande Avenue Paonia, CO 81428

**OPERATED BY:** USDA Forest Service, Grand Mesa, Uncompahgre and Gunnison National Forests

**INFORMATION:** (970) 527-4131; fs.usda.gov

**OPEN:** Mid-June–October

**SITES:** 11

**EACH SITE:** Picnic table, fire grate

**ASSIGNMENT:** First come, first served; no reservations

**REGISTRATION:** No registration

**FACILITIES:** Vault toilets, water

**PARKING:** At campsites only

**FEE:** $18 per night

**ELEVATION:** 9,600 feet

**RESTRICTIONS:** *Pets:* On leash only *Fires:* In fire grates only *Alcohol:* At campsites only *Vehicles:* 16 feet *Other:* 14-day stay limit

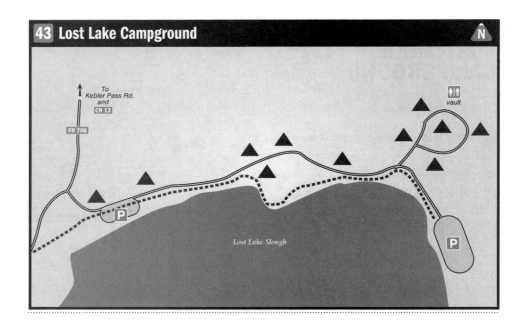

To Kebler Pass Rd. and CR 12

FR 706

vault

P

*Lost Lake Slough*

P

## GETTING THERE

From Paonia, drive north on CO 133 to CR 12 (Kebler Pass Road). The sign at the right turn will say "Crested Butte." Turn right on Kebler Pass Road and follow it for 16 miles to FS 706. Turn right on FS 706 and drive 2 more miles to Lost Lake Campground.

## GPS COORDINATES

**LATITUDE** N 38° 52' 9.8"
**LONGITUDE** W 107° 12' 33"

# 44
# LOST TRAIL
# CAMPGROUND

**S**OMETIMES A LONG DRIVE ON A dirt road ends in disappointment, but sometimes you are rewarded for enduring those bumpy, bouncy, dusty rides. In this case, you find Lost Trail Campground. Lost Trail sits in a beautiful valley surrounded on three sides by the San Juans, which form a horseshoe around the headwaters of the Rio Grande, which flow past your tent. Other peaks and crags stand out in bold relief. There are two outstanding hiking areas nearby and two fishing reservoirs close by as well.

The small campground with the big views has only seven campsites spread alongside lower Lost Creek just before its confluence with the Rio Grande. Mostly rockstrewn meadow, Lost Trail has some spruce and aspen that testify to the tough winters up here. The campsites are spread along a rocky road with a vehicle turnaround at the end. Enter the open campground and pass the first campsite on your right. It lies right alongside Lost Trail Creek and has the shade of some spruce. The next site is located in an especially rocky part of the meadow. The next campsite is opposite the creek and is in fullblown open terrain. The views? Simply outstanding. The shade? Nil.

Pass the hand-pump well and the pair of vault toilets for each gender, then come to the auto turnaround. The fifth site is down along the creek far away from the others. If you want privacy, stay here. The sixth site is on a rocky knoll in the center of the turnaround. A few aspens offer scant shade. The last site is away from the creek in the meadow and is another site with all view and no shade.

Don't worry too much about privacy—most people who drive this far are going to be like-minded tent campers who want to get way off the beaten track. It's axiomatic: The smaller the campground, the nicer campers are to one another. Come here and you'll probably make some new friends.

> *Lost Trail is the grandstand of the San Juan Mountains.*

## RATINGS

**Beauty:** ✩ ✩ ✩ ✩
**Privacy:** ✩ ✩ ✩
**Spaciousness:** ✩ ✩ ✩
**Quiet:** ✩ ✩ ✩ ✩
**Security:** ✩ ✩ ✩
**Cleanliness:** ✩ ✩ ✩

## KEY INFORMATION

**ADDRESS:** Lost Trail Campground Divide Ranger District Third and Creede Avenue Creede, CO 81130

**OPERATED BY:** USDA Forest Service, Divide Ranger District (Creede)

**INFORMATION:** (719) 658-2556; fs.usda.gov

**OPEN:** Mid-May–October

**SITES:** 7

**EACH SITE:** Picnic table, fire ring

**ASSIGNMENT:** First come, first served; no reservations

**REGISTRATION:** No registration

**FACILITIES:** Pump well, vault toilets

**PARKING:** At campsites only

**FEE:** No fee

**ELEVATION:** 9,500 feet

**RESTRICTIONS:** *Pets:* On leash only *Fires:* In fire rings only *Alcohol:* At campsites only *Vehicles:* 25 feet *Other:* 14-day stay limit

If (somehow) you tire of taking in the view from the campground, take a hike. The trail system around here is outstanding. The Lost Creek Trailhead is just a bit up the road. Here you can take the Lost Creek Trail up to Heart Lake or go toward the old mining area up toward the Continental Divide. About 30 minutes up the Lost Creek Trail will find you at the junction with the West Lost Creek Trail. Turn left here and come to a giant landslide caused by avalanche activity in 1991. A lake was formed from this event, and the Forest Service has stocked it. (And you thought new lakes were only created by man.)

The Continental Divide Trail is farther up Forest Service Road 520 near Stony Pass. This is the easy way to see the high country. The old Beartown mining site is off FS 520 on FS 506. Just down from the campground is the Ute Creek Trailhead. After fording the Rio Grande, you can access the Weminuche Wilderness along Ute Creek. This makes for an isolated fishing experience.

Two nearby reservoirs also offer fishing. Rio Grande Reservoir is closer, but harder to fish on unless you have a boat. It has more than 1,200 surface acres of trout water. Road Canyon Reservoir is a little farther away but is much better suited for bank fishing. It has only 140 surface acres, but the shoreline has a gentle grade, parking areas, and spots to put down a chair. The fishing is said to be good.

Bring all you will need to Lost Trail Campground. Supplies are limited in Creede, and you don't want to make an extra trip down that bumpy gravel road.

## GETTING THERE

From Creede, head west on CO 149 for 20 miles to FS 520 (Rio Grande Reservoir Road) and turn left. Follow FS 520 for 18 miles to Lost Trail Campground, which will be on your left.

## GPS COORDINATES

**Latitude** N 37° 46' 6.0"
**Longitude** W 107° 20' 57.0"

# 45
# MESA VERDE
# NATIONAL PARK:
## MOREFIELD CAMPGROUND

> *You'll need to stay at least one night at the largest campground in the national-park system to see the cliff dwellings and more at Mesa Verde.*

**Y**OU'VE GOT TO SEE MESA VERDE! The sight of the preserved remains of an extinct culture set into the inherent beauty of this park is one of Colorado's finest natural experiences. While driving on the park entrance road you are thinking about cliff dwellings and ancient cultures, but then you look over the Mancos Valley and San Juan scenery and realize that this place is special. The only extraordinary trait of the Morefield Campground is its size: more than 400 campsites. It is a pleasant enough place to stay and has adequate amenities to keep you from leaving the mesa, but the park itself has more than enough attractions to make you want to stay longer—the ranger-led tours, the view-laden hiking, good auto touring, and high-quality ranger programs every night.

The plethora of campsites are divided into nine loops and are spread out in a basin surrounded by ridges of trees and stone. In the basin, the primary vegetation is bushy Gambel oak with some occasional piñon pine. Each loop has comfort stations with flush toilets for each gender, combination water fountains/spigots, and a community sink area.

Pay your fee at the campground entry station and begin looking for a campsite. On the whole, campsite spaciousness is average; privacy depends on the amount of tree cover, which varies considerably. The forest's understory is generally grassy, with some sections of sage and brush. Navajo Loop is popular with tent campers. It is nestled in a hollow off to your left. The loop has many shaded sites and other sites that are exposed to the full sun, which can be tiresome on a long, summer day.

On down the way, Pueblo Road contains three loops and lots of campsites. This area is on a hill and has some piñon pines. The Zuni Loop is the best loop up here and has many good tent sites with a variety of sun and shade. There are good views across the basin of Prater Ridge.

## RATINGS

Beauty: ✿ ✿ ✿
Privacy: ✿ ✿
Spaciousness: ✿ ✿ ✿
Quiet: ✿ ✿ ✿
Security: ✿ ✿ ✿ ✿ ✿
Cleanliness: ✿ ✿ ✿ ✿ ✿

Stay away from the Ute Loop. It is the only loop with hookups and is the place of choice for RV campers. The Oraibi, Waipi, and Hano loops are all connected to one another. This area has many campsites that take a beating from the sun. The far views are good, but the near views of your fellow campers can be a little too close. The Apache Loop is sometimes closed until the campground begins to fill up. It is similar to the Oraibi loop.

Tent campers share Morefield Campground evenly with RV and pop-up campers. Morefield rarely fills and is fairly quiet, except for summer holidays, especially Memorial Day. A concessionaire offers showers and a laundry for a price. There is also a camp store, gift shop, cafe, and gas station. Snack bars are located at Chapin and Wetherill Mesas. Far View Lodge, located within the park, offers fine dining. You really can have it all!

Now, the reason why you came—to see the cliff dwellings. You must buy a ticket to go on a ranger-led tour of the three primary dwellings—Long House, Cliff Palace, and Balcony House. Each one was constructed in the 1200s by the ancestral Pueblos who made their lives atop the "Green Table." Cliff Palace has more than 150 rooms. The ranger leading the tours will satisfy your curiosity about each of the sites. You can tour the Spruce Tree House on your own. All-day and half-day concessionaire guided tours of the park leave Far View Lodge and Morefield Campground every morning. Mesa Verde is one place where it is smart to be led around by the nose. You'll want to ask many questions, and these rangers have all the answers.

First check out the park's visitor center and museum to get oriented after setting up camp. You'll come to the campground miles before the visitor center and museum. Make the Chapin Mesa driving tour and see the pit houses that came before the cliff dwellings. View other cliff dwellings from the road. The views of the landscape are exciting too.

Return to the campground to make the 1.5-mile walk out the Knife Edge to watch the sunset. And for the next day, there is Wetherill Mesa, Prater Ridge, the Cedar Tree Tower, and . . . this place will keep you busy. It is an all-inclusive affair. Bring your camera and a few free days, and have a fulfilling time.

| | |
|---|---|
| **ADDRESS:** | Mesa Verde National Park: Morefield Campground Aramark Mesa Verde Company P.O. Box 277 Mancos, CO 81328 |
| **OPERATED BY:** | Aramark Mesa Verde |
| **INFORMATION:** | (970) 564-4300 or (800) 449-2288; nps.gov/meve or visitmesaverde .com |
| **OPEN:** | Mid-April–October |
| **SITES:** | 435, some group sites |
| **EACH SITE:** | Picnic table, fire grate, tent pads |
| **ASSIGNMENT:** | First come, first served and by reservation |
| **REGISTRATION:** | At campground entry station |
| **FACILITIES:** | Water spigots, flush toilets, community dish sinks, phone (showers and laundry for fee from concessionaire) |
| **PARKING:** | At campsites only |
| **FEE:** | $23 per night tent sites, $33 per night RV sites, plus $10–15 park entrance fee, depending on season |
| **ELEVATION:** | 8,100 feet |
| **RESTRICTIONS:** | *Pets:* On leash only *Fires:* In fire grates only *Alcohol:* At campsites only *Vehicles:* 2 vehicles per site limit *Other:* 14-day stay limit |

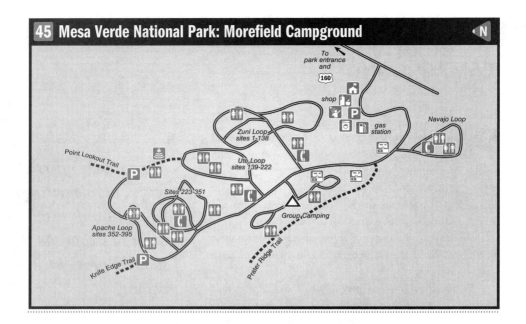

## GETTING THERE

From Cortez drive east on US 160 for 7.5 miles to the turnoff for Mesa Verde. Turn right and the Morefield Campground is 4 miles on your right.

## GPS COORDINATES

**LATITUDE** N 37° 11' 16"
**LONGITUDE** W 108° 29' 14"

**P**ERCHED ON THE WESTERN EDGE OF the Continental Divide, Mirror Lake reflects the snow and granite Rocky Mountains rimmed in verdant forests that colorfully contrast with the Colorado blue sky. Here you can come to escape the stress of modern civilization and reflect on the restorative qualities that a day, a week, or a weekend in our grand national forests can have on your attitude. Mirror Lake Campground is just such a place to seek your scenic respite.

While climbing sharply in your car along East Willow Creek, appreciate not only the beauty of the region but also the fact that you can access this high lake without having to walk all your supplies in. The road becomes very steep just before arriving at the lake. Make your right turn into the campground and climb another hill. Campsites appear to the left of the road in a stand of spruce, hidden from the water. Then you pop out on a small hill and the lake comes into view. The wind was calm on my visit, and the lake lived up to its name, reflecting Fitzpatrick Peak, Tincup Pass, and Emma Burr Mountain.

What was strange, though, was the state of the campground and lake—they were deserted. Such splendor with only me to appreciate it, although granted, it was a weekday. There were many favorable campsites as I drove through the loop. Several campsites were right on the lake, albeit a bit sun drenched. Others were set off in the woods with partial views of the lake. Though the amenities here are minimal (only vault toilets; you must bring your own water), the perk of easy access to an attractive, high lake right on the divide should attract more campers. The rough road and 16-foot vehicle length limit deter nearly all folks except for determined tent campers. Mirror Lake does get some weekend business, especially later in the summer. This same high elevation that lends such beauty also keeps campers from

> *Mirror Lake offers a restful alpine setting for tent campers who want to escape the summer heat of the valleys.*

## RATINGS

Beauty: ✩ ✩ ✩ ✩
Privacy: ✩ ✩ ✩
Spaciousness: ✩ ✩ ✩
Quiet: ✩ ✩ ✩ ✩
Security: ✩ ✩ ✩
Cleanliness: ✩ ✩ ✩

| | |
|---|---|
| ADDRESS: | Mirror Lake Campground Gunnison Ranger District 216 North Colorado Gunnison, CO 81230 |
| OPERATED BY: | USDA Forest Service, Grand Mesa, Uncompahgre, and Gunnison National Forests |
| INFORMATION: | (970) 641-0471; fs.usda.gov |
| OPEN: | Mid-June–October |
| SITES: | 10 |
| EACH SITE: | Picnic table, fire ring |
| ASSIGNMENT: | First come, first served; no reservations |
| REGISTRATION: | Self-registration on site |
| FACILITIES: | Vault toilets (no water) |
| PARKING: | At campsites only |
| FEE: | $10 per night |
| ELEVATION: | 11,000 feet |
| RESTRICTIONS: | *Pets:* On leash only *Fires:* In fire rings only *Alcohol:* At campsites only *Vehicles:* 16 feet *Other:* 14-day stay limit |

wandering up here in June because of the uncertainty of whether the campground is even open. Call ahead before you make the drive to Mirror Lake.

If you continue forward instead of veering right into the campground, you will come to the boat launch and parking area. The road that traces the left bank of the lake is the rough, four-wheel-drive road over 12,154-foot-high Tincup Pass. Only hand-propelled craft are allowed onto Mirror Lake. It keeps the peace that way. Mirror Lake encompasses 27 acres of clear water that harbors brook and rainbow trout. Forty percent of the bank is fishable; if you bring a kayak or canoe you can get to that other sixty percent of shoreline that everyone else misses.

Stream fishers can follow the outlet of Mirror Lake, East Willow Creek. Here, you can catch rainbow, brown, brook, or cutthroat trout. And if you follow East Willow Creek down, you'll come to the big water (and big fish) of Taylor Reservoir. The 2,000-acre lake offers the four fish species described above plus Kokanee salmon, lake trout, and pike. There are boat ramps here as well.

If you don't feel like fishing, take a walk. The four-wheel-drive road up to Tincup Pass is a couple of miles to the top and makes a great day hike. If you prefer, tramp a section of the Timberline Trail. The trailhead is a few hundred yards below the campground. This path generally follows the timber line north below the Sawatch Range. You can take the trail just a mile or so to Garden Basin and an old mine site, or you can walk all the way to Sanford Creek.

Mirror Lake may be best suited for getting an attitude adjustment in an alpine setting, a place to reflect on the really important things in life, like watching the sun set from the top of the Rockies.

## GETTING THERE

From Almont, drive north on FS 742 (Taylor Canyon Road) for 22 miles to Taylor Reservoir. Turn right at sign for Tincup on FS 765 and follow FS 765 for 8 miles to Tincup. In Tincup, turn left on FS 265 and follow it 3 miles to Mirror Lake.

## GPS COORDINATES

| | |
|---|---|
| **LATITUDE** | N 38° 44' 51" |
| **LONGITUDE** | W 106° 25'55" |

# RIDGWAY STATE PARK CAMPGROUND

> *This is one of the finest state parks in Colorado, if not the country.*

**O**NE OF THE NEWER **COLORADO STATE** parks, Ridgway is centered around a 1,000-surface-acre reservoir developed by the Bureau of Reclamation and run by the state of Colorado. This excellently designed recreational area integrates the best in human-made park facilities onto the natural features of the land. Two separate walk-in tent camper areas and three other quality campgrounds make this a must-stop for campers of all stripes.

The Dutch Charlie area features two campgrounds. The Dakota Terraces Campground is on lower, open terrain by the lake and has electrical hookups—this means RVs. The Elk Ridge Campground is high above the lake in a piñon-juniper forest. The views from Elk Ridge of the San Juan and Cimarron mountain ranges will blow your mind. There are two separate loops, both of which have electricity and a surprisingly high number of tent campers. But off Loop D is a set of ten walk-in tent campsites that will appeal to nearly every tent camper.

Walk the paved path that begins the tent-camper loop. The first campsite is handicapped accessible. Beyond that, the gravel path goes beneath some gnarled old piñons, with separate short paths leading to each well-separated site. Three of the sites are near the edge of a precipice over the lake. The mountain view is like a postcard landscape.

All sites have adequate shade trees, though high noon may present a heat problem. Large, level tent pads make for sound sleeping. Water spigots are located at the tent camper parking area. A modern restroom is nearby, though the showers and laundry are in the camper services building 100 or so yards distant.

Pa-Co-Chu-Puk Campground, 3.5 miles north of the Dutch Charlie area, has two loops that have water, bathrooms, and electricity, but they are out in the open and full of RVs. However, it also has a 15-site, walk-in tent camping loop that is across the Uncompahgre

## RATINGS

Beauty: ✩ ✩ ✩ ✩ ✩
Privacy: ✩ ✩ ✩
Spaciousness: ✩ ✩ ✩ ✩
Quiet: ✩ ✩ ✩ ✩
Security: ✩ ✩ ✩ ✩ ✩
Cleanliness: ✩ ✩ ✩ ✩ ✩

River from the rest of the park. This loop offers a rustic experience, yet is adjacent to the high-quality facilities that Ridgway offers. This loop is set in a ponderosa pine wood, complemented with Gambel oak and piñon pine, that gently rises up the slope of Log Hill Mesa.

Load your gear on a complimentary cart and bridge the river to the tenters' area. Campsites are snuggled here and there among the trees. The river is clearly audible. At each site, the picnic table and tent pads have been tastefully leveled, making your experience more comfortable, but still part of nature. Most of the sites are on the outside of the loop and are far from one another, making for a private and uncrowded experience. The water spigot is near the parking area and the showers are a good distance away, by the RV loops.

No matter where you are in this park, the first-rate facilities will make you wish all state parks had $22 million to spend on development. Recreating around here is first rate too. Ridgway Reservoir offers fishing for trout and Kokanee salmon. Waterskiing, parasailing, and riding wave runners are popular. No boat? No problem! The full-service marina will rent you anything from a canoe to a pontoon barge. A swimming beach and playground are ideal for family campers.

The Uncompahgre River flows below the reservoir. You can catch and release fish on the river or keep the fish caught on nearby ponds. Hikers have 15 miles of trails that course through the park to tramp. Four miles of trails are paved for inline skaters and bikers. Ranger-led hikes and programs inform campers about the natural resources of Ridgway. Make sure and check out the visitor center too. The Dallas Creek Recreation Site is at the south end of the park. Here, you can hike and fish along the reservoir and also head up Dallas Creek over the pedestrian bridge.

You would think such a fantastic state park would be constantly full. Not so. However, it does get busy around the major holidays and later in the summer. But I have it on the park manager's word that September is the time to visit Ridgway. Be sure to put this gem of a state park on your to-do list.

| | |
|---|---|
| **ADDRESS:** | Ridgway S. P. 28555 US 550 Ridgway, CO 81432 |
| **OPERATED BY:** | Colorado State Parks |
| **INFORMATION:** | (970) 626-5822; parks.state.co.us |
| **OPEN:** | Mid-April– September |
| **SITES:** | 25 walk-in tent-only sites, 255 other |
| **EACH SITE:** | Tent-only has tent pad, fire grate, grill, picnic table; others also have water and electricity |
| **ASSIGNMENT:** | By reservation or pick an available site on arrival |
| **REGISTRATION:** | By phone (call (800) 678-CAMP (2267) or (303) 470-1144 in Denver) or reserveamerica.com |
| **FACILITIES:** | Hot showers, flush toilets, laundry, phone, vending machines |
| **PARKING:** | At campsites or walk-in tent campers' parking area |
| **FEE:** | $7 Parks Pass plus $16–18 per night walk-in tent site, $24–26 others |
| **ELEVATION:** | 7,000 feet Elk Ridge, 6,600 feet Pa-Co-Chu-Puk |
| **RESTRICTIONS:** | *Pets:* On leash only *Fires:* In fire rings only *Alcohol:* 3.2% beer only *Vehicles:* On paved roads only *Other:* 14-day stay limit |

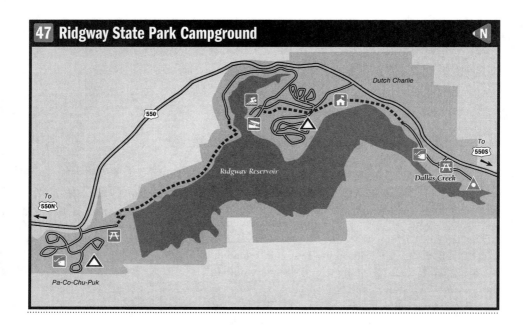

## 47 Ridgway State Park Campground

## GETTING THERE

From Ridgway, drive north on US 550 for 5 miles to the Dutch Charlie entrance of the park, which will be on your left.

## GPS COORDINATES

**LATITUDE** N 38° 12' 28.0"
**LONGITUDE** W 107° 44' 3.8"

# 48
# SILVER JACK
# CAMPGROUND

**S**ILVER JACK CAMPGROUND IS ARGUABLY ONE of the
prettiest campgrounds in one of the prettiest spots
in Colorado. Located near the forks of the Cimarron
River in the shadow of Uncompahgre Peak, the campground borders 2-mile-long Silver Jack Reservoir,
which enhances the forests, meadows, and summits
of the nearby Uncompahgre Wilderness. Only hand-
propelled boats are allowed on the reservoir, maintaining peace and quiet to go along with the scenery both in
and beyond the campground.

> *Stay among the aspens at the Uncompahgre National Forest's finest campground.*

The campground is situated on a knoll above the
lake, surrounded by aspens. Their leaves flutter in the
wind, emitting a purr and creating an ever-changing
mosaic of light on the forest floor. Tall grass forms an
unbroken understory that contrasts with the white trunks
of the aspen. This is the reason you come tent camping
to begin with.

Silver Jack has three tiered loops. The roads are
paved, along with each camper's parking spot, which
really cuts down on the dust. The first loop, Ouray, has
a short two-way road with campsites along it before
the actual loop starts. Ouray is at the lowest level and
has 20 campsites set in the aspens. One small meadow
breaks up the trees, along with a very occasional small
evergreen.

The Chipeta Loop circles around a meadow of its
own. Yet all the campsites are in an extremely dense
aspen wood. The young trees make for shady campsites
and offer great privacy, especially on the upper section
of this loop. This seems to be the most popular place
to camp.

The Sapinero Loop is the highest on the knoll and is
sometimes closed until the campground fills. However,
it is my favorite loop. Here, the aspens are older, larger,
and allow more light to form a more flowery understory.
You can also see the surrounding mountains better.

## RATINGS

Beauty: ✿ ✿ ✿ ✿ ✿
Privacy: ✿ ✿ ✿ ✿
Spaciousness: ✿ ✿ ✿
Quiet: ✿ ✿ ✿ ✿
Security: ✿ ✿ ✿ ✿
Cleanliness: ✿ ✿ ✿ ✿ ✿

## KEY INFORMATION

**ADDRESS:** Silver Jack
Campground
Ouray Ranger
District
2505 South
Townsend
Montrose, CO
81402

**OPERATED BY:** USDA Forest
Service, Grand
Mesa,
Uncompahgre,
and Gunnison
National Forests

**INFORMATION:** (970) 240-5300;
fs.usda.gov

**OPEN:** Memorial Day–
September

**SITES:** 60

**EACH SITE:** Picnic table,
fire grate

**ASSIGNMENT:** First come,
first served;
no reservations

**REGISTRATION:** Self-registration
on site

**FACILITIES:** Water spigots,
vault toilets

**PARKING:** At campsites only

**FEE:** $14 per night

**ELEVATION:** 8,900 feet

**RESTRICTIONS:** *Pets:* On leash only
*Fires:* In fire grates
only
*Alcohol:* At camp-
sites only
*Vehicles:* 30 feet
*Other:* 14-day
stay limit

The road rolls upward with campsites spread far apart, though they tighten up as the loop is completed.

Water spigots and vault toilets are evenly spread about the campground. There should be no trouble finding a campsite in June, when the weather is less predictable and can still be chilly. But in July and August, arrive early to ensure a campsite on weekends. September is a great time to visit and watch the aspen leaves change color. Any time is a great time to relax in this wonderful campground setting.

Of course, you may want to get active. Hiking, fishing, and boating are the main activities here. An informal trail circles Silver Jack Reservoir, so you can bank-fish for rainbow trout, brook trout, and Kokanee salmon. By all means, if you have a canoe, bring it. Your arms are the only motor you can use here. The scenery from a boat in the middle of the lake is inspiring. You won't care if you catch fish or not.

Fly fishers like to try their luck on one of the three forks of the Cimarron River, as the waters tumble down from the wilderness above. Beaver Lake lies a mile below Silver Jack and is also popular for fishing. The smaller Fish Creek reservoirs are just a few miles north of Silver Jack on Cimarron Road. No one swims in these chilly lakes.

Silver Jack derived its moniker from the mine of the same name located in the Uncompahgre Wilderness just south of the campground. You can hike up the East Fork Trail (228) to the old mine site. Always be careful near any mine, closed or open. Beyond the mine site are two waterfalls of the East Fork.

You don't have to go to Europe to climb the Matterhorn. There's one right here in the Uncompahgre Wilderness. Take the Middle Fork Trail (227) for a challenging day hike to top the 13,590-foot peak. Uncompahgre Peak is a fourteener, but it can't be reached in one day from this side of the wilderness.

For an easier hike, go to Cimarron Ridge, across the reservoir. It can be accessed from Trail 222. You'll end up at 10,800-foot Lou Creek Pass, overlooking your camping paradise. Or hike up to High Mesa on the Alpine Trail, which starts near the campground. Or you may just want to hang out and watch the aspens flutter in the wind.

## GETTING THERE

From Montrose, drive 23 miles east on US 50 to Cimarron Road. Turn right on Cimarron Road and follow it 21 miles to Silver Jack, which will be on your right.

## GPS COORDINATES

**LATITUDE** N 38° 14' 2.9"
**LONGITUDE** W 107° 32' 17"

> *Stone Cellar is in the heart of 15,000-acre Saguache Park, the largest meadowland in the entire national forest system.*

**W**HEN YOU CROSS THE **C**ONTINENTAL **D**IVIDE at South Pass, Saguache (pronounced suh-WACH) Park opens up before you. It is an expanse of rolling, grassy terrain cut with creeks and bordered by massive peaks fringed in forest land. Smaller, lesser-used forest roads splinter off in all directions, beckoning you to see what lies over the next hill. Farther down, along the Middle Fork of Saguache Creek, lies the Stone Cellar Campground. Beyond the campground, open park land rolls on to the La Garita Mountains and the La Garita Wilderness.

The wilderness looks over (La Garita means "the lookout") more meadowlands, as well as old-growth forests and trout-laden streams and lakes. There are more than 120,000 acres and 175 miles of trails to enjoy in this seldom visited slice of wild Colorado. The Wheeler Geologic Area is also within the wilderness. Rock spires, pinnacles, domes, and other stone oddities emerge from the earth.

When you drop down to the campground, you will immediately notice a lack of trees. That's only appropriate because the campground is in Saguache Park. It took a few minutes for me to get used to the openness, but I began to appreciate the scenery: Middle Fork flowing out of a meadow from above into a canyon down below, vertical rock walls rising up at the campground, and the views of the distant mountains.

A wooden stock fence surrounds three of the campsites here. There is one campsite outside the fence a few yards away, toward the head of the meadow on a forest road. This site must either be for campers who have been bad or for campers who love cows, since livestock graze in Saguache Park.

The other three sites border the creek. One site is off to the right and is farthest away from the rock walls. This will avail more views, but less shade. The other

## RATINGS

**Beauty:** ✿ ✿ ✿ ✿
**Privacy:** ✿ ✿
**Spaciousness:** ✿ ✿ ✿ ✿
**Quiet:** ✿ ✿ ✿ ✿
**Security:** ✿ ✿
**Cleanliness:** ✿ ✿ ✿

two campsites are downstream in a very green, grassy meadow, between a granite wall and the clear, gurgling water. It is a short walk to these campsites from the parking area. A vault toilet and pump well are conveniently set in the middle for all campers, except the site outside the stock fence.

Anyone here should be a tent camper, because if it rains, the road back to CO 114 will be very slick. You shouldn't have a problem unless you are towing something, like a pop-up trailer. If you want to come to Saguache Park but can't stand the thought of camping in the open, several forest roads in the area lead to wooded camp locations. Saguache Park deserves a visit, especially later in the summer when the whole place is awash in wildflowers.

If you do drive the roads around here, make sure to take the marked road to Chimney Rocks. However, to explore the La Garita Wilderness, you must abandon your vehicle and take to your feet. The land is high and the trails start high, then lead even higher.

Farther up Forest Service Road 787 beyond the campground is the South Saguache Trail. It starts at 10,400 feet and follows the creek for good fishing and easy access to the high country toward Half Moon Pass. Whale Creek Trail starts here too and heads toward Palmer Mesa.

FS 744, which turns off right before the campground and has the one lonesome campsite, leads farther up the Middle Fork of Saguache Creek to another trailhead. Here you can walk to the headwaters of the Saguache and into lake country. Half Moon Pass Trail starts here too. It is a 7-mile, one-way hike to the Wheeler Geologic Area, but it can be done in a single day. If you leave early in the morning, you will have time to view the area and still return by nightfall.

The North Fork Saguache has its own trail to headwaters made up of several small tributaries; a few beaver ponds are scattered along the way. This trail is outside the wilderness and can be accessed by FS 776. Walk around or drive around, either way you will get an eyeful at Saguache Park.

## KEY INFORMATION

**ADDRESS:** Stone Cellar Campground Saguache Ranger District 46525 CO 114 Saguache, CO 81149

**OPERATED BY:** USDA Forest Service, Rio Grande National Forest

**INFORMATION:** (719) 655-2547; fs.usda.gov

**OPEN:** Memorial Day–Labor Day

**SITES:** 5

**EACH SITE:** Picnic table, fire ring

**ASSIGNMENT:** First come, first served; no reservations

**REGISTRATION:** No registration

**FACILITIES:** Pump well water, vault toilets

**PARKING:** At campsites only

**FEE:** $7 per night

**ELEVATION:** 9,500 feet

**RESTRICTIONS:** *Pets:* On leash only *Fires:* In fire rings only *Alcohol:* At campsites only *Vehicles:* 25 feet *Other:* 14-day stay limit

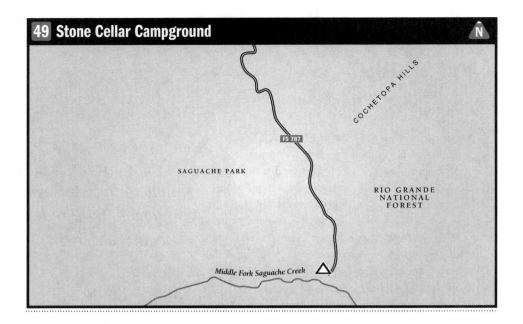

## GETTING THERE

From Saguache, head west on CO 114 and follow it 22 miles to FS 804 (Archuleta Creek Road). Turn left on FS 804 and follow it 4 miles to CR NN14. Turn left on CR NN14 and follow it for 0.8 mile to FS 787. Turn right on FS 787 and follow it 13 miles to Stone Cellar Campground.

## GPS COORDINATES

**Latitude** N 38° 1' 12.3"
**Longitude** W 106° 40' 42"

**T**RANSFER **P**ARK IS STEEPED IN HISTORY. The attractive, mountain-rimmed meadow was once a point where tools and supplies were transferred from horse-drawn wagons to mules for use beyond the rugged Florida River canyon in the late 1800s. Ore, mostly gold and silver, would be brought down in the wagons. These days, the 11-acre site is such a scenic campground that it just may prevent you from enjoying the hiking, fishing, rafting, train riding, and town touring that the area has to offer.

Drop into the upper meadow and come to the campground. Miller Mountain stands guard over Transfer Park. There are two camping loops. The right-hand loop has ten campsites and is set in a mature aspen grove mixed with some Ponderosa pine, Douglas fir, and small clearings. Smaller trees and brush form a fairly thick understory. The campsites are large and well separated from one another. Wooden posts delineate the sites from one another. The forest closes near the meadow, then opens back up as the loop is completed. You can find just about any combination of sun and shade you desire. There is one vault toilet and one spigot in the center of the loop.

The left-hand loop is lower and closer to the Florida River. Drop down along Transfer Park and the 15 campsites begin. The forest here is more mixed conifers and thus is shadier. The thicker forest and rock outcrops make for a closed-in, intimate feeling on this loop. The gush of the Florida River can be heard loud and clear. About half the campsites are on the heavily wooded inside of the loop. A few campsites border the river gorge, but a wood fence prevents campers from falling into the river below. Two vault toilets and two water spigots serve this loop.

This campground used to be on a reservation basis, but was taken off because it did not fill. Forest Service

> *Make a transfer to the most attractive campground in the San Juan National Forest.*

## RATINGS

Beauty: ☆ ☆ ☆ ☆ ☆
Privacy: ☆ ☆ ☆ ☆
Spaciousness: ☆ ☆ ☆ ☆
Quiet: ☆ ☆ ☆ ☆
Security: ☆ ☆ ☆
Cleanliness: ☆ ☆ ☆ ☆

## KEY INFORMATION

| | |
|---|---|
| **ADDRESS:** | Transfer Park Columbine East Ranger District 367 South Pearl St. Bayfield, CO 81122 |
| **OPERATED BY:** | USDA Forest Service, San Juan National Forest |
| **INFORMATION:** | (970) 884-2512; fs.usda.gov |
| **OPEN:** | Mid-May–Labor Day |
| **SITES:** | 25 |
| **EACH SITE:** | Picnic table, fire grate |
| **ASSIGNMENT:** | First come, first served; no reservations |
| **REGISTRATION:** | Self-registration on site |
| **FACILITIES:** | Water spigot, vault toilets, trash pick-up |
| **PARKING:** | At campsites only |
| **FEE:** | $17 per night |
| **ELEVATION:** | 8,600 feet |
| **RESTRICTIONS:** | *Pets:* On leash only *Fires:* In fire grates only *Alcohol:* At campsites only *Vehicles:* 26 feet *Other:* 14-day stay limit |

personnel say it is rarely at over 50 percent capacity—an odd fact, but a good one, for tent campers who find their way to this gorgeous place.

Those who do make it here now have to choose among the array of nearby activities. You can trace the old mine trail up along the Florida River. It is primarily used now by fishermen who vie for native cutthroat trout and a few Kokanee salmon, which make their way up from Lemon Reservoir. Hiking comes naturally, as the Burnt Timber Trail starts at the top of the campground. This path leads into the nearly 500,000-acre Weminuche Wilderness. A reasonable destination is the southern end of Lime Mesa.

Just up bumpy Forest Service Road 597, which starts by Florida Campground, are two short hikes into Lost Lake and Stump Lake. Lost Lake has no fish. A longer trek goes up Endlich Mesa to the City Reservoir area, which is more attractive than it sounds. Downstream from Transfer Park is Lemon Reservoir. It is a rainbow trout, kokanee salmon, and pike fishery. The popular angling areas are near the dam and at the Lemon Day Use Area.

The rest of the action is down Durango way. It is a historic western town that is cashing in on the tourism craze. The historic district is real, and you can find anything you desire to consume or own. However, if you want to move through some good natural scenery, try the narrow-gauge Silverton Train or a rafting trip on the Piedre or Animas Rivers.

The Durango and Silverton Railroad was constructed in the 1880s to haul gold and silver from the San Juan Mountains. The train trip is an easy way to see the Weminuche Wilderness. It is an all-day affair getting to and from Silverton, but it will be one of the more scenic trips of your life.

The rivers offer more rollicking action. The lower Animas goes through Durango and is a little on the tame side. But the Upper Animas offers Class IV to V rapids. The Piedre has Class III to IV rapids and a wild atmosphere. Contact one of the many outfitters listed at the Durango Chamber of Commerce.

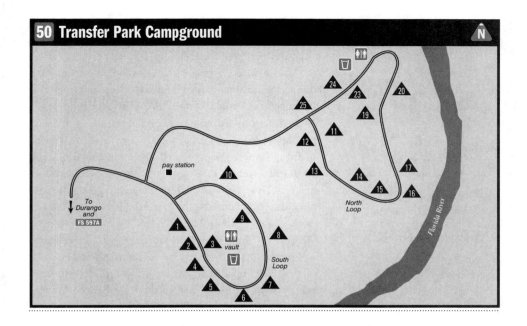

## GETTING THERE

From Durango, take CR 240 (Florida Road) north for 14 miles to CR 243. Stay left on CR 243, going for 5 miles, passing Lemon Reservoir, to FS 597A. Turn left on FS 597A and veer left again after crossing the Florida River. Stay right while passing through Florida Campground and come to Transfer Park in 1 mile.

## GPS COORDINATES

| | |
|---|---|
| **LATITUDE** | N 37° 27' 46.3" |
| **LONGITUDE** | W 107° 40' 47" |

# APPENDIXES & INDEX

# APPENDIX A: CAMPING EQUIPMENT CHECKLIST

Except for the large and bulky items on this list, we keep a plastic storage container full of the essentials for car camping so they're ready to go when we are. We make a last-minute check of the inventory, resupply anything that's low or missing, and away we go.

## COOKING UTENSILS

Bottle opener

Bottles of salt, pepper, spices, sugar, coffee, tea, and cooking oil and maple syrup in waterproof, spillproof containers

Can opener

Corkscrew

Cups, plastic or tin

Dish soap (biodegradable), sponge, and towel

Flatware

Food of your choice

Frying pan, spatula

Fuel for stove

Ice

Lighter, matches in waterproof container

Plates

Pocketknife

Fire starter

Pot with lid

Stove

Tin foil

Wooden spoon

## FIRST-AID KIT

Aspirin

Band-Aids

First aid cream

Gauze pads

Insect repellent

Moleskin

Sunscreen/lip balm

Tape, waterproof adhesive

## SLEEPING GEAR

Pillow

Sleeping bag

Sleeping pad, inflatable or insulated

Tent with ground tarp and rainfly

## MISCELLANEOUS

Bath soap (biodegradable), washcloth, towel

Camp chair

Candles

Cooler

Deck of cards

Flashlight/headlamp

Paper towels and toilet paper

Plastic zip-top bags

Shovel

Sunglasses

Warm clothes, raingear, hiking boots

Water bottle

Wool blanket

## OPTIONAL

Backpack for hiking

Barbecue grill

Binoculars

Cell phone

Compass

Field guides on bird, plant, and wildlife identification

Fishing rod and tackle

GPS

Lantern

Maps (road, trail, topographic, etc.)

Reading material

# APPENDIX B: CONTACT INFORMATION

## U.S. BUREAU OF LAND MANAGEMENT

**BIG DOMINGUEZ CAMPGROUND**
2815 H Road
Grand Junction, CO 81506
(970) 244-3000
co.blm.gov/gjra/dominguezcg.htm

**LITTLE SNAKE BLM FIELD OFFICE**
455 Emerson Street
Craig, CO 81625
(970) 826-5087 or (970) 826-5000;
co.blm.gov/lsra/camping.htm

## COLORADO STATE PARKS

**ARKANSAS HEADWATER RECREATION AREA**
307 West Sackett Avenue, P.O. Box 126
Salida, CO 81201
(719) 539-7289; parks.state.co.us

**BONNY LAKE STATE PARK**
30010 County Road 3
Idalia, CO 80735
(970) 354-7306; parks.state.co.us
bonny.lake.park@state.co.us;
Bonny marina and store: (970) 354-7339

**COLORADO STATE FOREST**
2746 Jackson County Road 41
Walden, CO 80480
(970) 723-8366; parks.state.co.us;
state_forest@state.co.us

**GOLDEN GATE CANYON STATE PARK**
92 Crawford Gulch Road
Golden, CO 80403
(303) 582-3707 or (303) 642-3856 in
summer; parks.state.co.us
golden.gate.park@state.co.us

**JACKSON LAKE STATE PARK**
26363 CR 3
Orchard, CO 80649
(970) 645-2551; parks.state.co.us
jackson.lake@state.co.us

**MUELLER STATE PARK CAMPGROUND**
P.O. Box 39
Divide, CO 80814
(719) 687-2366; parks.state.co.us
mueller.park@state.co.us

**RIDGWAY STATE PARK**
28555 Highway 550
Ridgway, CO 81432
(970) 626-5822; parks.state.co.us

**RIFLE FALLS STATE PARK CAMPGROUND**
00050 Road 219
Rifle, CO 81650; (970) 625-1607
parks.state.co.us; rifle.gap.park@state.co.us

**STEAMBOAT LAKE STATE PARK
CAMPGROUND**
Box 750; Clark, CO 80428
(970) 879-3922; parks.state.co.us/
steamboat; steamboat@state.co.us

**LARIMER COUNTY PARKS AND OPEN
LANDS DEPARTMENT**
1800 South County Road 31
Loveland, CO 80537
970) 679-4570
larimer.org/parks

## NATIONAL PARK SERVICE

**COLORADO NATIONAL MONUMENT**
Fruita, CO 81521
(970) 858-3617; nps.gov/colm

**CURECANTI NATIONAL RECREATION AREA**
102 Elk Creek
Gunnison, CO 81230
(970) 641-2337 ext. 205; nps.gov/cure

**DINOSAUR NATIONAL MONUMENT**
4545 East Highway 40
Dinosaur, CO 81610-9724
(970) 374-3000 or (435) 781-7700;
nps.gov/dino

## NATIONAL PARK SERVICE (CONTINUED)

GREAT SAND DUNES NATIONAL MONUMENT
11999 Highway 150
Mosca, CO 81146
(719) 378-2312; nps.gov/grsa

NORTH RIM CAMPGROUND
102 Elk Creek
Gunnison, CO 81230
(970) 641-2337; nps.gov/blca

ROCKY MOUNTAIN NATIONAL PARK
Estes Park, CO 80517
(970) 586-1206; nps.gov/romo

## USDA FOREST SERVICE

ARAPAHO AND ROOSEVELT NATIONAL FORESTS
Pawnee National Grassland
Boulder Ranger District
2140 Yarmouth Avenue
Boulder, CO 80301
(303) 541-2500; fs.fed.us/r2/arnf

CANYON LAKES RANGER DISTRICT
2150 Centre Avenue, Building E
Fort Collins, CO 80526
(970) 295-6700; fs.fed.us/r2/arnf

PAWNEE NATIONAL GRASSLAND
660 'O' Street
Greeley, CO 80631
(970) 346-5000; fs.fed.us.r2/arnf

SULPHUR RANGER DISTRICT
9 Ten Mile Drive, P.O. Box 10
Granby, CO 80446
(970) 887-4100

DIVIDE RANGER DISTRICT
3rd and Creede Avenue
Creede, CO 81130
(719) 658-2556; fs.fed.us/r2/riogrande

GRAND MESA, UNCOMPAHGRE, AND GUNNISON NATIONAL FORESTS
Grand Valley Ranger District
277 Crossroads Boulevard, Suite A
Grand Junction, CO 81506
(970) 242-8211; fs.fed.us/r2/gmug

GUNNISON RANGER DISTRICT
216 North Colorado
Gunnison, CO 81230
(970) 641-0471; fs.fed.us/r2/gmug

OURAY RANGER DISTRICT
2505 South Townsend
Montrose, CO 81402
(970) 240-5300; fs.fed.us/r2/gmug

PAONIA RANGER DISTRICT
P.O. Box 1030
North Rio Grande Avenue
Paonia, CO 81428
(970) 527-4131; fs.fed.us/r2/gmug

MEDICINE BOW–ROUTT NATIONAL FORESTS, THUNDER BASIN NATIONAL GRASSLAND
Yampa Ranger District
P.O. Box 7, 300 Roselawn Avenue
Yampa, CO 80483
(970) 638-4516; fs.fed.us/r2/mbr

PIKE AND SAN ISABEL NATIONAL FORESTS, CIMARRON AND COMANCHE NATIONAL GRASSLANDS
Grand Valley Ranger District
325 West Rainbow Boulevard
Salida, CO 81201
(970) 242-8211; fs.fed.us/r2/psicc/sal

LEADVILLE RANGER DISTRICT
810 Front Street
Leadville, CO 80461
(719) 486-0749
fs.fed.us/r2/psicc/leadville

**SAN CARLOS RANGER DISTRICT**
3170 East Main Street
Cañon City, CO 81212
(719) 269-8500;
fs.fed.us/r2/psicc/sanc

**SOUTH PLATTE RANGER DISTRICT**
19316 Goddard Ranch Court
Morrison, CO 80465
(303) 275-5610; fs.fed.us/r2/psicc/spl

**RIO GRANDE NATIONAL FOREST**
Cathedral Campground
Divide Ranger District
13308 West Highway 160
Del Norte, CO 81132
(719) 657-3321; fs.fed.us/r2/riogrande

**CONEJOS PEAK RANGER DISTRICT**
15571 County Road T-5
La Jara, CO 81140
(719) 274-8971; fs.fed.us/r2/riogrande

**SAGUACHE RANGER DISTRICT**
46525 CO 114
Saguache, CO 81149
(719) 655-2547; fs.fed.us/r2/riogrande

**SAN JUAN NATIONAL FOREST**
Mancos-Dolores Ranger District
100 North 6th Street
Dolores, CO 81323
(970) 882-7296; fs.fed.us/r2/sanjuan

**PAGOSA RANGER DISTRICT**
108 Second Street
Pagosa Springs, CO 81147
(970) 264-2268; fs.fed.us/r2/sanjuan

**TRANSFER PARK COLUMBINE EAST RANGER DISTRICT**
367 South Pearl Street
Bayfield, CO 81122
(970) 884-2512; fs.fed.us/r2/sanjuan

**WHITE RIVER NATIONAL FOREST**
Blanco Ranger District
317 East Market Street
Meeker, CO 81641
(970) 878-4039
fs.fed.us/r2/whiteriver

**EAGLE RANGER DISTRICT**
P.O. Box 720, 125 West Fifth Street
Eagle, CO 81631
(970) 328-6388
fs.fed.us/r2/whiteriver

**HOLY CROSS RANGER DISTRICT**
24747 US 24
Minturn, CO 81645
(970) 827-5715; wildernet.com

# INDEX

BEST
TENT
CAMPING
COLORADO

**DEAR CUSTOMERS AND FRIENDS,**

**SUPPORTING YOUR INTEREST IN OUTDOOR ADVENTURE,** travel, and an active lifestyle is central to our operations, from the authors we choose to the locations we detail to the way we design our books. Menasha Ridge Press was incorporated in 1982 by a group of veteran outdoorsmen and professional outfitters. For many years now, we've specialized in creating books that benefit the outdoors enthusiast.

Almost immediately, Menasha Ridge Press earned a reputation for revolutionizing outdoors- and travel-guidebook publishing. For such activities as canoeing, kayaking, hiking, backpacking, and mountain biking, we established new standards of quality that transformed the whole genre, resulting in outdoor-recreation guides of great sophistication and solid content. Menasha Ridge continues to be outdoor publishing's greatest innovator.

The folks at Menasha Ridge Press are as at home on a white-water river or mountain trail as they are editing a manuscript. The books we build for you are the best they can be, because we're responding to your needs. Plus, we use and depend on them ourselves.

We look forward to seeing you on the river or the trail. If you'd like to contact us directly, join in at www.trekalong.com or visit us at www.menasharidge.com. We thank you for your interest in our books and the natural world around us all.

**SAFE TRAVELS,**

*Bob Sehlinger*

**BOB SEHLINGER**
**PUBLISHER**